Color Atlas of
Histopathology

G. Austin Gresham

TD, MD, ScD, MA, FRCPath.

Fellow of Jesus College, Cambridge
Professor of Morbid Anatomy and Histopathology
Home Office Pathologist
United Kingdom

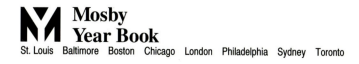

**Mosby
Year Book**

St. Louis Baltimore Boston Chicago London Philadelphia Sydney Toronto

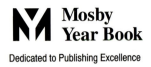

Mosby–Year Book, Inc.
11830 Westline Drive
St. Louis, MO 63146

English edition published as *A Colour Atlas of General Pathology,* Second Edition, in
1992 (first edition published in 1971) by Wolfe Publishing, an imprint of Mosby–Year
Book Europe Limited, 2–16 Torrington Place, London WC1E 7LT, UK.

Library of Congress Cataloging-in-Publication Data.
Gresham, G. A. (Geoffrey Austin)
    Color atlas of histopathology / G. Austin Gresham. -- 2nd
 ed.
     p. cm.
    Includes index.
    ISBN 0-8151-3989-6
    1. Pathology, Histological--Atlases. Pathology--Atlases.
 I. Title.
    [DNLM: 1. Pathology -- atlases. QZ 17 G831c]
RB33.G74 1993
611'.018--dc20
DNLM/DLC
for Library of Congress
                                             92-8480
                                               CIP

Contents

To my family

Preface

Pathology is the science of disease. It is concerned with the causes of disease or disorder and the effects of disease-producing agents upon living things, both plants and animals. The ultimate aim of many people who study pathology is the prevention and cure of the disease, but first we must study disease as an entity in itself. Only in this way, without the impelling demand to avoid or to treat, can we start impartially to discover mechanisms in the disease-producing process.

This atlas is about disease processes, that is, the various events that appear as disease occurs and progresses. It shows pictures of various tissue and cellular responses to injurious agents. The idea is to lay a foundation of knowledge about the fundamental responses that are common to many disorders. When the student has mastered the basic responses he or she will find no difficulty in understanding special disorders in various systems of the body. For example, inflammation is a basic reaction of many living things to injury of various sorts and, whatever the cause of the inflammation, the response and the mechanisms responsible are fundamentally the same.

This, then, is an atlas of general rather than special pathology and is prepared for medical students and other students of biology. Many medical schools now teach basic general pathology to students in the preclinical years. This book should be of assistance to them. General pathology is also part of the training of medical laboratory technicians in histopathology and they will find the book useful.

A mole with fungus disease of its lungs is as interesting as a cow with tuberculosis or a person with stomach cancer: each is a living thing responding to injury. Such patterns of response to injury are the subject of our studies in this book.

Acknowledgements

I am indebted to my colleagues in the Department who provided me with material and especially to our photographer Chris Burton who took many of the pictures. Susan Green deciphered my writing, typed the script and did an excellent job.

1 Examination of sections

Most of the work that is done in general pathology is concerned with thin, stained sections of tissue rather than with a study of whole organs. The majority are stained with haematoxylin (blue) and eosin (red) (H and E); occasionally, other stains help to elucidate the nature of the process (special stains).

It is important to have a regular routine for the examination of sections. First, look with a hand lens and make a low power drawing. This indicates the need to study different parts of the section. Then turn to the microscope. Most of the useful information can be derived from study with a low power objective. Higher power lenses are generally less useful, except for a study of cell detail.

Having studied the section, write a description of it. Whether you can interpret your findings or not is immaterial at this stage. First, learn to observe thoroughly and accurately: diagnosis will then come easily and automatically.

1–4 show a partly dead (necrotic) pituitary and illustrate the diagnostic sequence.

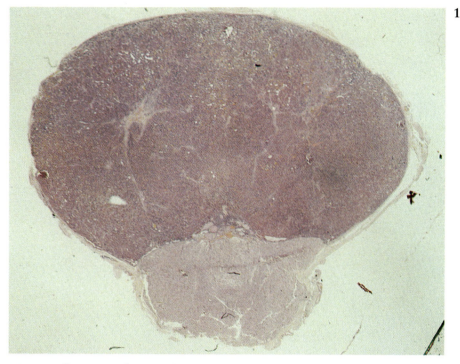

1

1 A normal pituitary showing the pars anterior, stained purple, at the top. The pars nervosa is the paler, smaller part below. (*H and E*)

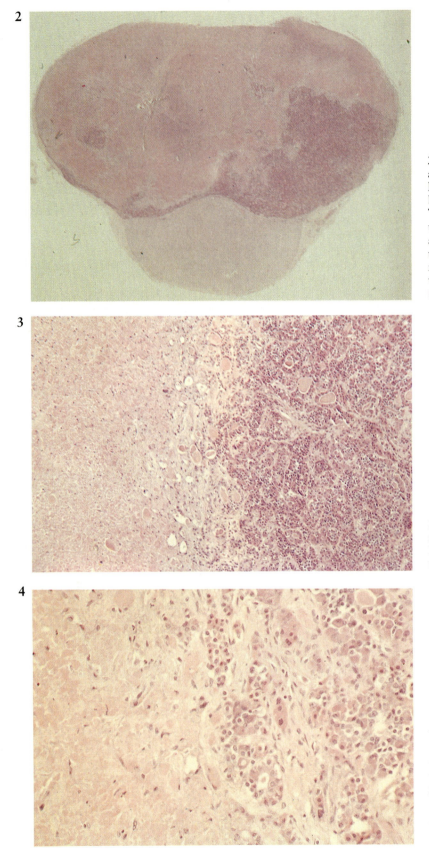

2 Pituitary necrosis. The necrotic area is in the anterior lobe on the left. Surviving cells are seen at the bottom right in the anterior lobe. This is the view that can be obtained using a hand lens. It is a good plan always to look first with a lens and then to examine with higher power microscope objectives later. In this way no part of the section is missed. (*H and E*)

3 Normal pituitary on the right, necrotic (dead) pituitary on the left. Note the lack of nuclear staining in the necrotic part. (*H and E × 4*)

4 Necrotic pituitary on the left, with a normal anterior pituitary on the right, high power view. Note the nuclei of connective tissue cells that have survived in the necrotic area. They are less specialised cells and less vulnerable to ischaemia (q.v.) than the glandular cells of the pituitary. (*H and E × 10*)

2 The lesion

It is convenient to have a general term to describe anything that is wrong with a living thing. The term we use is 'lesion', which literally means 'a hurting'. So we call a fracture of the skull a lesion, a boil on the skin a lesion, a tumour of the bone a lesion, and so on. Lesions are often seen with the naked eye: they are then said to be macroscopic. Further elucidation of their nature can only be obtained when a thin section is examined under the microscope. Most of this atlas is about the microscopic appearances of lesions, for only in this way can the precise mechanism of causation be determined. 5 and 6 illustrate a scar in the heart muscle and show the macroscopic and microscopic appearances.

Macroscopical and microscopical views of a lesion

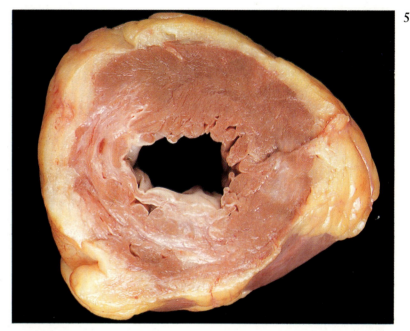

5

5 Macroscopic view of a slice taken through the apex of the heart. The pericardium is fatty, the muscle is brown. Within the muscle (mainly to the left) are grey-white areas of fibrous scarring caused by narrowed coronary arteries producing myocardial ischaemia (q.v.).

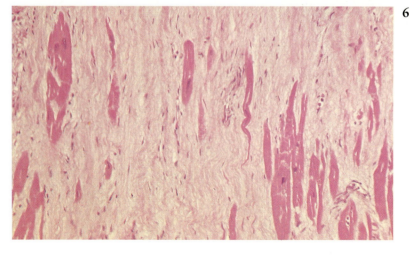

6

6 Pink heart muscle fibres set in a pale pink fibrous background. This is a scar in the myocardium. Only a few heart muscle fibres have survived the ischaemic process. (*H and E × 4*)

Survival of less specialised cells in infarction

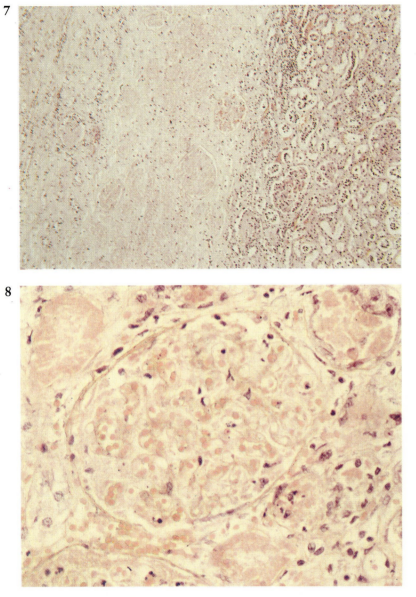

7 Kidney showing dead (necrotic) tissue on the left and surviving tissue on the right. This is the edge of a renal infarct (q.v.) caused by obstruction of an artery to the necrotic area of the kidney. (*H and E × 4*)

8 Kidney showing a higher power view of an infarct. The glomerulus and tubules contain pink necrotic cells. The less specialised spindle-shaped connective tissue cells have retained their nuclear staining. (*H and E × 20*)

3 The normal cell and tissue

Cellular structure

Mammalian cells are enormously variable in shape, size and appearance, and it is therefore not surprising that diseased cells vary considerably. Yet there are certain features common to many cells, for example, most cells have mitochondria and these are very sensitive to any agent, except viruses, that may damage the cells. Mitochondrial damage, therefore, is an early event in cellular disorder. Another general feature is that epithelial cells tend to be rather more vulnerable than mesodermal cells. If we look at the edge of a renal infarct (this being an area of necrosis produced by vascular obstruction) we can see dead epithelial cells and surviving fibroblasts of the connective tissue that have withstood the ischaemia (4, 7, 8).

Basement membranes and reticulin

An important feature of many epithelial cells is the basement membrane (9, 10). This supports the cell and also contributes to cellular nutrition. Basement membranes are made of a gelatinous matrix of polysaccharide (mucosubstance) that stains readily with the periodic acid-Schiff (PAS) method. Reticulin fibres are embedded in the matrix; these fibres are chemically similar to collagen but differ in periodicity when seen by electron microscopy (2.7 nm as against 6.4 nm). They also differ from collagen in being argentaffin, that is, they take up silver salts and are stained black by a deposition of metallic silver on them. Reticulin patterns are especially important in the diagnostic histopathology of the lymph nodes and liver (11, 12). A disturbance of the pattern, as we shall see later, is an early indication of disease in these organs.

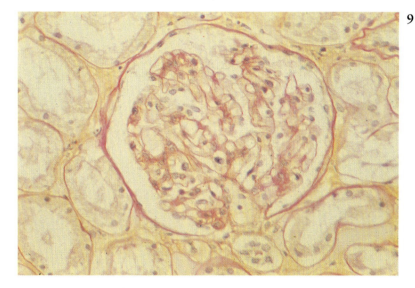

9

9 **Normal glomerulus.** The capillary and tubular basement membranes are stained pink by the periodic acid-Schiff method. This demonstrates the carbohydrate component of the basement membrane. (*PAS × 20*)

10

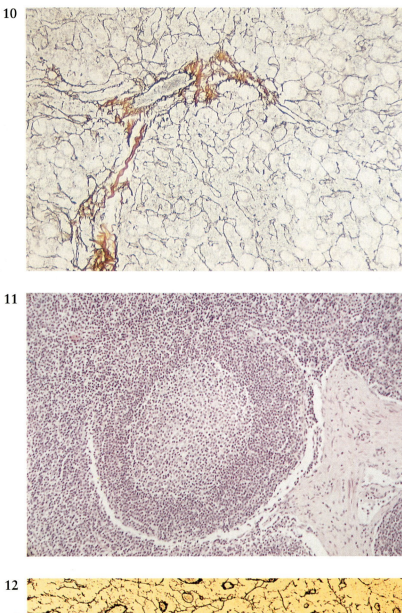

10 Basement membranes of liver cells stained black by a silver method. The individual liver cells cannot be seen. With this method collagen fibres in the portal tracts stain brown. (*Gordon and Sweet × 20*)

11

11 Reactive centre in the cortex of a lymph node (also called a germinal centre). Note central macrophages and peripheral layers of lymphocytes. (*H and E × 20*)

12

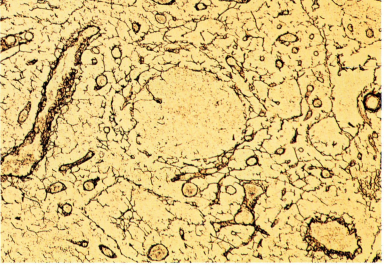

12 Reactive centre showing few reticulin fibres. The black fibres around the centre are supporting sinusoids and blood vessels. This is a normal pattern which is disturbed in neoplastic (q.v.) involvement of lymph nodes. (*Gordon and Sweet × 10*)

Electron microscopy

The basic ingredients of a cell are shown in the diagram of an electron photomicrograph (**13**). There are many variations upon this basic theme. The plasma membrane is thrown into folds (microvilli) in those cells, like jejunal and renal proximal tubular cells, that are concerned with absorption. Protein-making cells, like plasma cells (q.v.), have a rich endoplasmic reticulum studded with ribosomes. Energetic cells have contractile myofilaments or, in the case of axons of some nerve cells, are electrically insulated with coils of myelin. Most cells contain mitochondria and these are vulnerable to all sorts of injury except by viruses; they are the first of the cell organelles to show signs of damage. Lysosomes are bags of hydrolytic enzymes that cause the cell to digest itself (autolysis) or digest other particles (phagocytosis).

Electron microscopy has illuminated the study of cellular disorder mainly by linking organelles with particular functions. This enables the histopathologist to translate morphological alterations into functional disturbances. In some diseases, for example, renal glomerular disorders, the only changes that can be detected are demonstrable by the electron microscope, since the alterations are far too slight to be seen by light microscopy (**14, 15**).

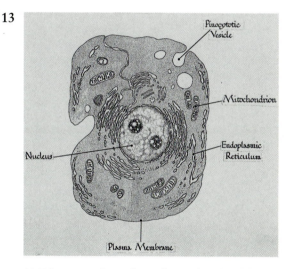

13 Diagram of a cell as shown by the electron microscope.

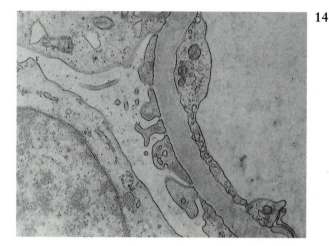

14 Normal glomerulus as shown by electron microscopy. Normal foot processes in the central gap. (× *15,000*)

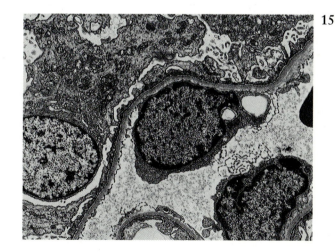

15 Fusion of foot processes in a glomerulus (top centre). This 'minimal change' disease is not visible by light microscopy and can be seen only by the electron microscope. (× *15,000*)

Cellular chemistry

Histochemistry

After ordinary light microscopy, histochemistry is the method most often used for the elucidation of pathological processes. It is an attempt to identify the chemical constituents of tissue by using staining methods that have a clearly defined chemical basis. The earliest of these methods was Perls' for haemosiderin, where ferric iron in the tissue combines with potassium ferrocyanide to form Prussian blue (16, 17).

A variety of histochemical methods are used to show mucin in cells, and other polysaccharides in connective tissues. Methods for polysaccharides (mucosubstances) are numerous, but not all have a clearly defined basis, like Perls' method for ferric iron.

Mucopolysaccharides (mucosubstances) are stained by such dyes as mucicarmine and alcian blue, and are also coloured by the PAS method and by Hale's method (18–20). In Hale's method, colloidal iron is made to react with the sulphonic group of the acid mucopolysaccharide, and the fixed iron is then demonstrated by Perls' method.

Enzymes in cells and tissues are also demonstrable by histochemical methods. The tissue slice or section is incubated with a substrate; the enzyme then acts on the substrate and liberates a component that is made visible in the section by forming either a coloured compound or an insoluble precipitate. For example, alkaline phosphatase is shown by treating a section with glycerophosphate. The liberated phosphate is then treated with cobalt nitrate to produce cobalt phosphate that is finally converted to cobalt sulphide. So the presence of the enzyme is indicated by a black precipitate over and around the cells (21, 22).

16

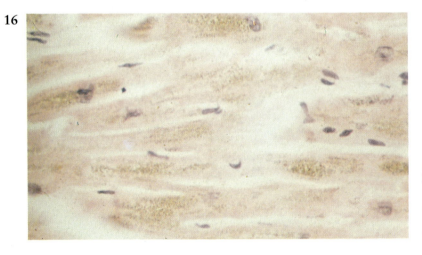

16 Heart muscle showing brown haemosiderin in the fibres. This is seen in haemochromatosis where iron is absorbed in excess from the gut and deposited in many tissues including heart muscle. (*H and E × 20*)

17

17 Heart muscle. The same tissue as 16 stained by Perls' method. This shows blue staining ferric iron in the heart muscle fibres. (*Perls' × 20*)

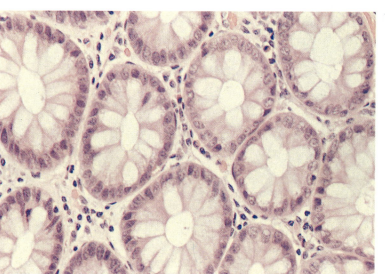

18 A transverse section of colonic **mucosa** showing cellular spaces that contain mucin. (*H and E × 20*)

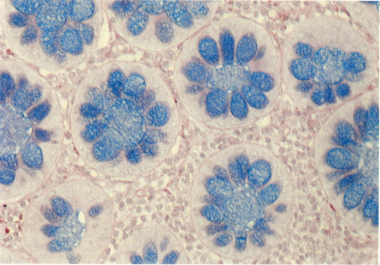

19 A transverse section of colonic **mucosa** showing mucin staining blue with Alcian blue, and basement membranes staining magenta with the periodic acid-Schiff method. (*Alcian blue, PAS × 20*)

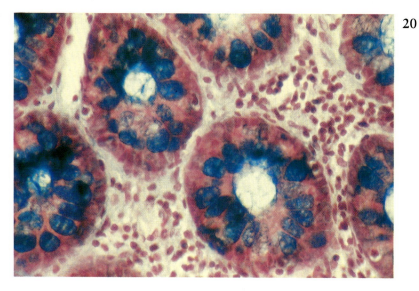

20 **Colonic glands** stained by Hale's method. The mucin is a deep blue colour. (*Hale's method × 40*)

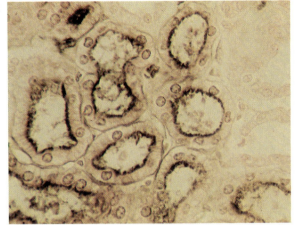

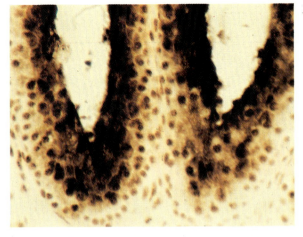

21 Section of a preen gland from a bird. Cells lining the glandular spaces have a black internal border, due to the presence of alkaline phosphatase. (*Gomori's method × 10*)

22 Black alkaline phosphatase in the renal tubules of a rat. (*Gomori's method × 40*)

Fluorescence microscopy and immunochemistry

There are other modifications of light microscopy which are being used with increasing frequency in histopathology. Briefly, fluorescence depends upon either the fact that some tissue components fluoresce naturally in ultraviolet light (primary fluorescence), or the fact that certain components can be made to fluoresce by treating a section with certain dyes called fluorochromes (secondary fluorescence). Primary fluorescence is shown by elastic fibres after formalin fixation: they are ice-blue when viewed with a microscope using ultraviolet illumination. Fluorochromes are widely used, for example, the *Mycobacterium tuberculosis* fluoresces yellow after treatment with auramine O (**128**). Because these organisms are often difficult to find in sections or in sputum, secondary fluorescence is a valuable, rapid way of detecting them when they are present in small numbers. Antibodies can be made fluorescent, and when applied to a section they can detect such things as immunoglobulins (**23**).

Tetracycline is fluorescent, and because it is taken up by growing bone it can, when fed to an animal, be subsequently detected in sections of bone viewed in ultraviolet light. Yellow areas of tetracycline fluorescence reveal areas of new bone formation, and this is a useful technique in the study of bone diseases (**24, 25**).

The discovery of monoclonal antibodies which react specifically with particular cellular components has revolutionised modern histochemistry. The presence of intermediate filaments, such as desmin and vimentin, can be detected with precision, and epithelial cell membranes can be clearly outlined (**26**). Immunochemistry has proved especially valuable in studies of neoplasms (q.v.) of lymphoid tissues. Monoclonal antibodies also enable the main type of B and T lymphocytes and their various subsets to be recognised. Ability to recognise different sorts of lymphoid neoplasms by these methods is of value in assessing their prognosis, and in evaluating treatment. Some neoplasms (q.v.) are so poorly differentiated (q.v.) that their precise origin can be defined only by immunochemical stains or by electron microscopy.

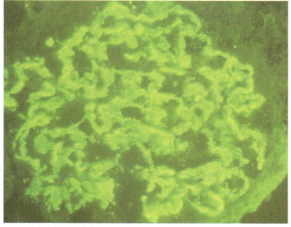

23 A renal glomerulus fluorescing bright green. The green material is deposits of immunoglobulin in the basement membranes. From a case of glomerulonephritis. (× 40)

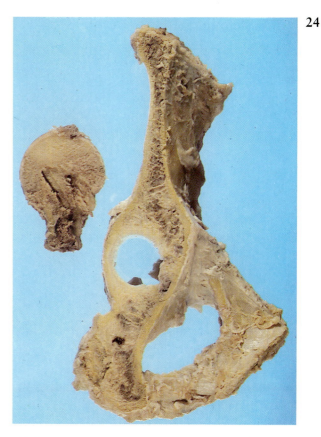

24 An innominate bone and the head of a humerus. Note the faint yellow tinge to the bone due to accumulated tetracycline.

25 Tetracycline fluoresces yellow in ultraviolet light.

26 Epithelial cell cytoplasm outlined in brown. This has been stained with an antibody generated against epithelial cell cytokeratin. (*Immunoperoxidase × 40*)

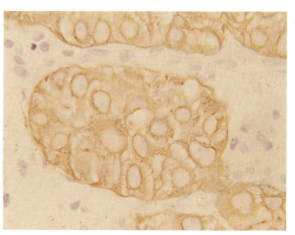

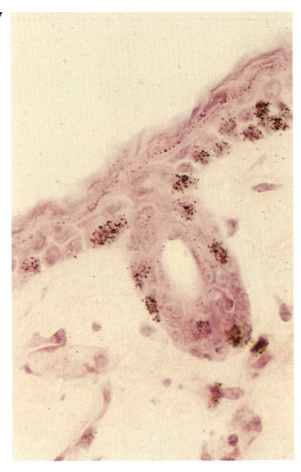

27

Cells take up various elements and compounds and incorporate them into their structure. If these substances are radioactive isotopes, then their presence within the cell can be shown by autoradiography. Some examples are thyroid cells that take up ^{131}I, dividing cells of all sorts that take up tritiated thymidine, and connective tissue cells that incorporate ^{35}S in order to make the mucopolysaccharide matrix.

If an animal is given tritiated thymidine it is taken into cells that are about to divide. If a section of the tissue is then taken and coated with photographic emulsion, the cells that contain the label are covered with black dots of silver. This is caused by the radiation from the cells precipitating silver from the photographic emulsion. Hence the mitotic rate can be found (27).

27 Rat skin. The black dots are nuclei that have taken up tritiated thymidine. They have been shown by exposing a photographic film over the section. (*Autoradiography × 40*)

Cellular variation

Cell types

Cells differ in shape, size, number and distribution or organelles and, of course, in their response to disease-producing agents. The three following examples illustrate such differences.

Nerve cells have abundant RNA (Nissl substance) in their cytoplasm. Loss of this is an early feature of nerve cell damage and is called chromatolysis. This change is reversible when the noxious stimulus is removed (28, 29).

Plasma cells are protein synthetic lymphoid cells and have, in consequence, abundant endoplasmic reticulum. When they are very active, as in many chronic inflammations (q.v.), they form intra and extracellular aggregates of antibody (Russell bodies) (30–32).

Mesothelial cells are flat pavement type cells that are barely visible in a transverse section, but when some noxious agent injures the surface, such as the pleura or peritoneum, the cells swell up and become almost cuboidal in shape. A similar change occurs in synovial cells in many joint conditions. These cells are barely visible in the normal state, but any irritation within the joint causes them to swell and become conspicuous (33, 34).

A few examples of the ways in which cells alter in disease are given below. We shall study many more subsequently.

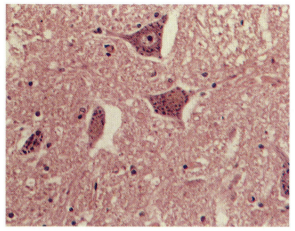

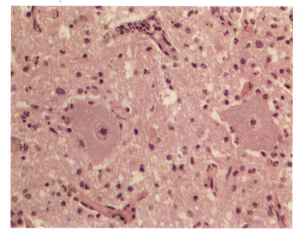

28 A cluster of normal motor neurons in the anterior horn of the spinal cord. Note the abundant clumps of dark staining Nissl substance of the cytoplasm of the cells. (*H and E × 10*)

29 Pale staining neurons that have lost their Nissl substance (chromatolysis). From the spinal cord of a case of poliomyelitis. (*H and E × 20*)

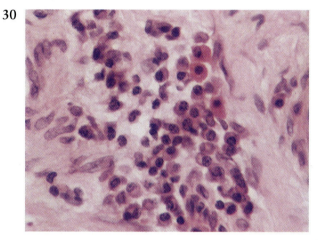

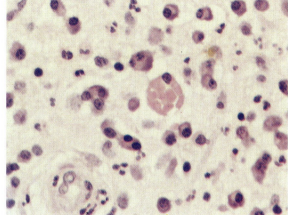

30 Plasma cells with the characteristic 'clock face' arrangement of nucleoprotein, eccentric nuclei and vacuolate cytoplasm. A few cells around the middle of the section have abundant red cytoplasm: these are mast cells. (*H and E × 40*)

31 Russell bodies. The pink globular bodies in the central cells are Russell bodies. There are also many adjacent plasma cells. (*H and E × 40*)

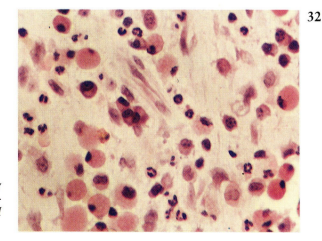

32 Groups of red staining Russell bodies. The intensity of red staining is variable (**31**). Most of the Russell bodies are found within the cytoplasm of plasma cells. (*H and E × 40*)

33

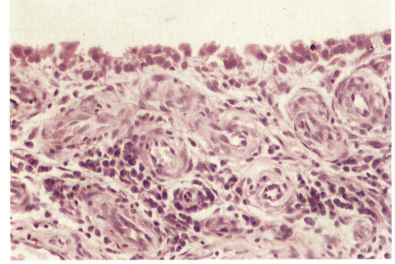

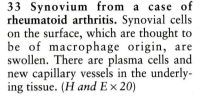

33 **Synovium from a case of rheumatoid arthritis.** Synovial cells on the surface, which are thought to be of macrophage origin, are swollen. There are plasma cells and new capillary vessels in the underlying tissue. (*H and E × 20*)

34

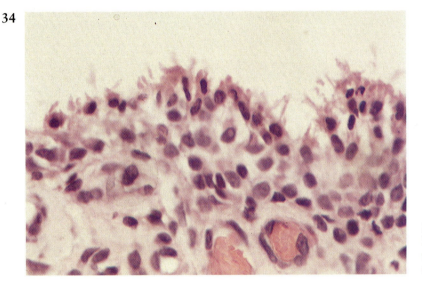

34 **Enlarged 'irritated' synovial cells.** Note the characteristic surface granules that appear in many joint disorders. (*H and E × 40*)

Atrophy

Atrophy is the shrinkage of cells. It may be physiological, as in the shrinking uterus after pregnancy or in the mammary lobules after lactation. It also occurs in old age, or in certain diseases associated with great loss of weight: the heart shrinks, and the fibres become atrophic and contain much brown pigment (called lipochrome, because of its lipid content, or 'wear and tear' pigment). This pigment is also seen in certain neurons, in liver and in other cells, and is probably derived from fragmented mitochondrial membranes (35–39).

Atrophy is caused by hypoxia, by disuse of a structure such as a limb, or by injurious agents.

For example, atrophy of the villi of the small gut is sometimes due to the ingestion of gluten (from bread) in the diet. Such atrophy leads to failure of fat absorption and the production of bulky frothy stools (steatorrhoea). When gluten is removed from the diet the small gut mucosa may return to normal. Gluten enteropathy (sometimes called coeliac disease) is due to sensitivity to gliaden. This is reflected by the large numbers of lymphocytes between the epithelial cells of the small gut in this condition (40–42).

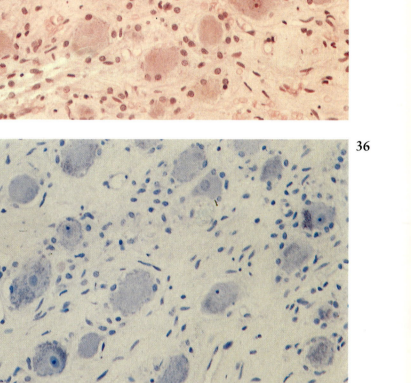

35 Autonomic ganglion cells containing brown lipochrome pigment in the cytoplasm. (*H and E × 20*)

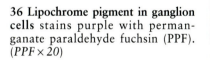

36 Lipochrome pigment in ganglion cells stains purple with permanganate paraldehyde fuchsin (PPF). (*PPF × 20*)

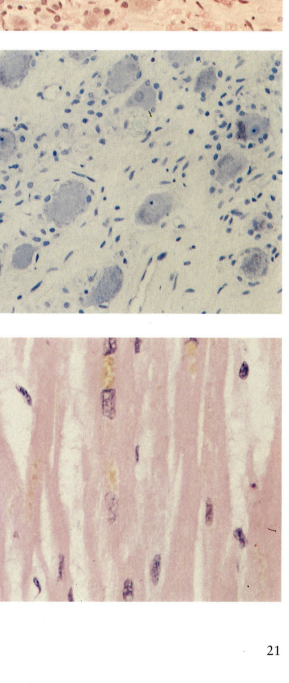

37 Heart muscle fibres containing yellow lipochrome pigment, often situated at the poles of the nuclei. (*H and E × 40*)

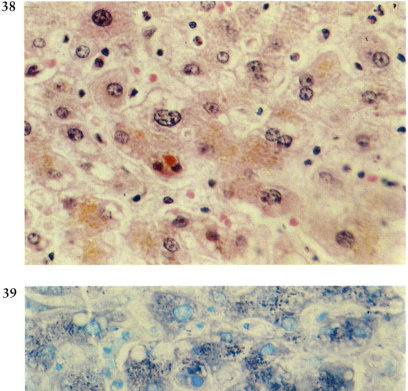

38 Liver cells contain lipochrome pigment. Rounded clumps of bile pigment are present in the canaliculi. (*H and E × 40*)

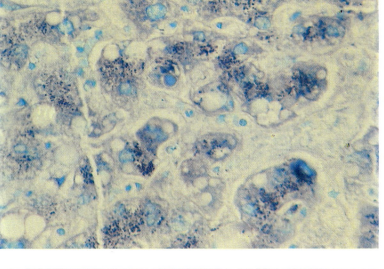

39 Atrophy. Lipochrome pigment stains purple with permanganate paraldehyde fuchsin. Bile pigment stains light blue as do cell nuclei. (*PPF × 40*)

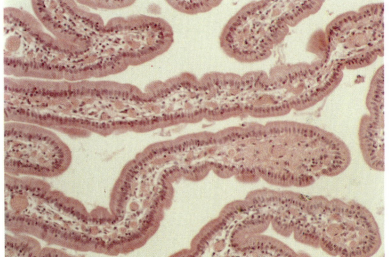

40 Normal jejunal villi are long and slender. Only occasionally can one see lymphocytes in the epithelial layer. (*H and E × 10*)

41

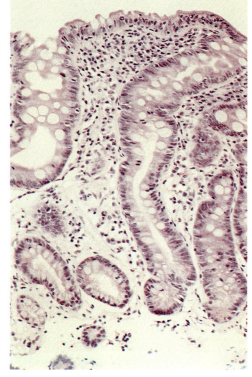

41 Jejunal mucosa from a case of gluten dependent enteropathy. The villi have disappeared, the mucosal surface is flat, and the glandular crypts are elongated. Lymphocytes are seen in the epithelium, and plasma cells in the lamina propria. (*H and E × 10*)

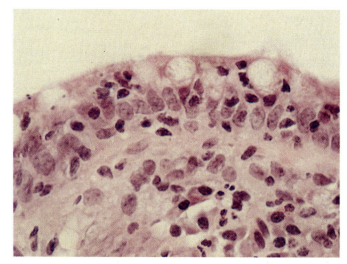

42

42 Jejunum. Lymphocytes are seen within the epithelial cell layer of the jejunum. Plasma cells are present in the lamina propria. (*H and E × 40*)

Hypertrophy

This term can be applied to both cells and organs. Hypertrophy of an organ is a symmetrical increase in size; hypertrophy of a cell is a uniform increase in the size of the nucleus and cytoplasm. When the organ is required to do more work, the cells hypertrophy. This is readily seen in the myometrial cells of the pregnant uterus, and it also occurs in left ventricular myocardial fibres when the arterial blood pressure rises, as in hypertensive disease (**43–45**). Unfortunately, hypertrophy is not always accompanied by an increase in blood supply to the enlarged cell. This can be seen in the myocardium; as the fibres get large, they become relatively short of blood supply (ischaemia), and they then atrophy and are replaced by fibrous tissue.

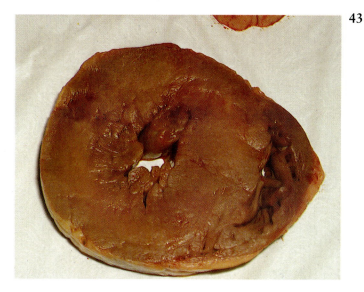

43

43 Hypertrophy. A transverse slice through the apex of the heart of a hypertensive person. The left ventricle on the left side of the picture is greatly hypertrophied (thickened).

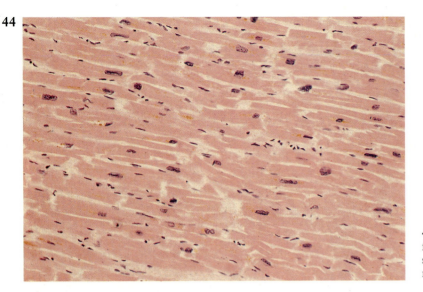

44 Hypertrophy. Low power view from a hypertensive left ventricle showing irregular enlargement of myocardial fibres. (*H and E × 10*)

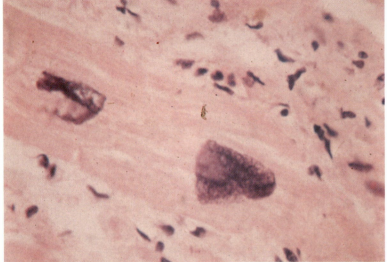

45 High power view of hypertrophied fibres. Not only do the fibres enlarge, but the nuclei increase in size as well. (*H and E × 40*)

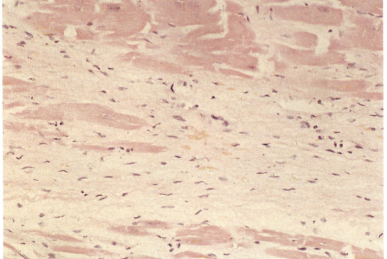

46 Irregular hypertrophy of myocardial fibres adjacent to a myocardial scar. Note the lipochrome pigment in the scar. This is all that remains of myocardial fibres that have perished. (*H and E × 10*)

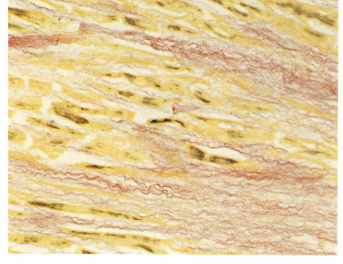

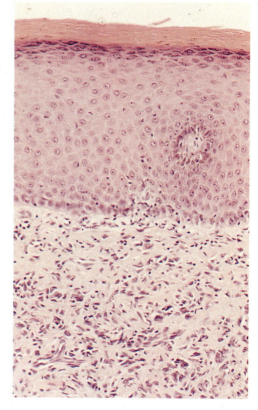

47 Myocardial fibres. Strands of pink scar tissue separating myocardial fibres stained yellow. Note the irregular hypertrophy of the fibres. (*Weigert's resorcin fuchsin ponceau S × 10*)

48 Thickening of the epidermis over a benign tumour of the dermis (dermatofibroma q.v.). This hypertrophic reaction of the epidermis occurs over many benign skin tumours, and consists of thickening of the stratum corneum (hyperkeratosis) and of the cellular epidermis. (*H and E × 10*)

Hyperplasia

This is an increase in the number of cells in a tissue. Hyperplasia is a physiological event in the breast during pregnancy; the cells multiply in order to prepare for lactation after delivery. A similar hyperplasia occurs in the endometrial cells during the menstrual cycle. Hyperplasia is also a pathological process, for example, it can occur in the prostate of elderly men, causing the organ to hypertrophy or enlarge. It also occurs as a result of high oestrogen levels in elderly women, where the cells lining the endometrial glands increase greatly in numbers and size: in other words, there is both hyperplasia and hypertrophy of the cells (**49, 50**). Hyperplasia of cells lining the alveoli of the lung is another example of pathological hyperplasia. This phenomenon is called the 'epithelialisation' of the alveoli, and is the end result of a wide variety of chronic (long-standing) insults that damage lung tissue. It is, for example, a feature of chronic lung infections (**51**).

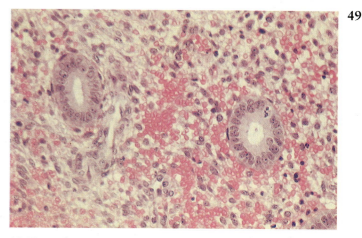

49 Normal non-secretory endometrial tubules. Note the single layer of epithelial cells. (*H and E × 4*)

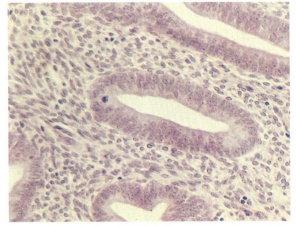

50 Endometrial tubules lined by cell layers more than one cell thick. The cell nuclei are enlarged. From an elderly woman with hyperoestrogenism. (*H and E × 10*)

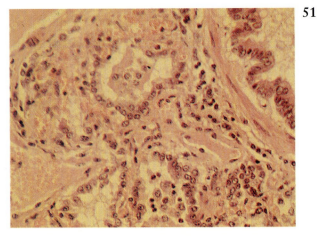

51 Hyperplasia. Section of lung showing a bronchiole on the right. Alveoli in the middle of the picture are lined by plump Type 2 pneumocytes. This is a common reaction to many causes of lung disease. (*H and E × 20*)

Metaplasia

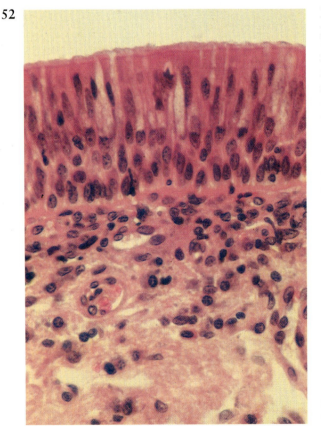

Metaplasia is a change in cell character. For example, the transformation of ciliated cells in the bronchi into squamous cells is called squamous metaplasia (**52–54**). It is usually the result of repeated chronic irritation such as smoking, and may be the precursor of carcinoma (q.v.). Similar squamous metaplasia occurs in the transitional epithelium of the urinary tract, and is caused by irritating hydrocarbons excreted in the urine.

Hormones will sometimes change the character of an epithelium, for example, squamous metaplasia in the prostate can be caused by stilboestrol (a synthetic oestrogen), which is used for the treatment of prostatic carcinoma (q.v.) (**55–56**).

52 Pseudostratified epithelium of the bronchus. There is an excess of lymphocytes and of plasma cells in the subepithelial layer. (*H and E × 40*)

53

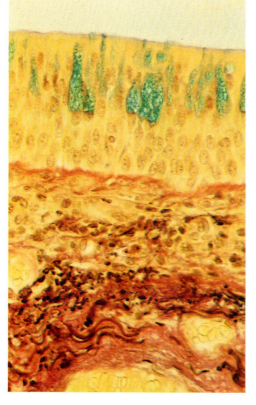

53 Mucus secreting cells in bronchial epithelium, stained green. (*Alcian blue × 40*)

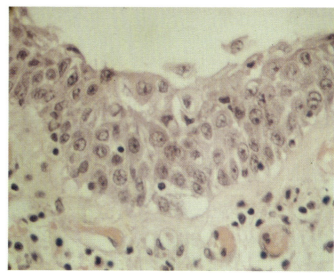

54

54 Squamous metaplasia of bronchial epithelium. The epithelium has lost the cilia and mucus producing cells, and has been transformed into a layer of cells resembling the squamous cells of the epidermis. This is a common reaction to irritants such as tobacco smoke. (*H and E × 20*)

55

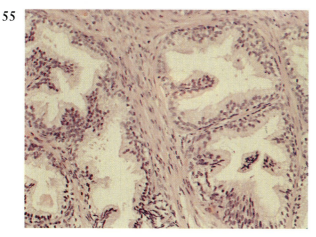

56

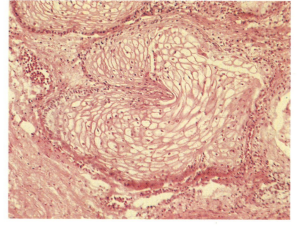

55 Section of normal prostate. The acini are lined by columnar cells and separated by a fibrous and muscular stroma. (*H and E × 10*)

56 An enlarged prostatic acinus filled with squamous cells. This form of metaplasia occurs in men treated with oestrogens for prostatic carcinoma. (*H and E × 20*)

4 Cellular damage

Cell swelling

Cellular swelling is the earliest evidence of cellular injury; this is because the mitochondria are very vulnerable to noxious agents. When the mitochondria are damaged, the cellular metabolism fails, leading to sodium ions entering the cell; this, and the osmotic effect caused by the breakdown of large macromolecules within the damaged cell, causes cloudy swelling. This change is reversible and precedes the other changes described in this chapter. Macroscopically, the organ affected by cloudy swelling is heavier than normal, has a featureless cut surface, and bulges from the capsule (for example, the liver and kidney) (57). Microscopically, the cells are swollen and finely granular, the granules being bits of mitochondria and other structural proteins (58).

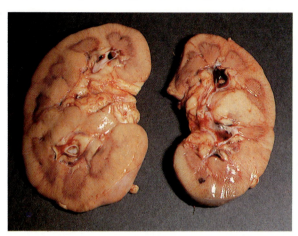

57

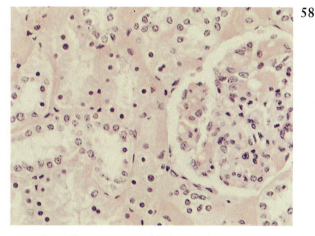

58

57 Cell swelling. Swollen, pale cut surfaces of kidney, showing cloudy swelling. The cortex and interpyramidal columns are greatly swollen, due to post mortem breakdown of tubular epithelial cells.

58 Cell swelling. Section of kidney. The glomerulus is fairly well preserved. Convoluted tubular epithelial cells are swollen and fragmented, due to post mortem autolysis. (*H and E × 20*)

Cell vacuolation

Cloudy swelling is the first step of cellular degeneration; the next phase is the appearance of vacuoles in the cytoplasm of the damaged cell; subsequently the cell may die and undergo necrosis. As we have said already, the effects of noxious agents often follow this pattern, but do vary according to:

- The *type* of cell affected.
- The *nature* of the noxious stimulus.
- The *intensity* of the stimulus.
- The *duration* of the stimulus.

Considering the type of cell, vacuolation of liver cells is usually due to accumulation of fat, the so-called fatty change. Vacuolation of renal tubular cells is due to the collection of watery fluid in the cells, the so-called hydropic change. Both types of vacuolation are reversible processes. The fatty change in the liver can be due to a variety of noxae:

- Hypoxia, e.g. anaemia.
- Poisons, e.g. alcohol.
- Metabolic disorder, e.g. diabetes mellitus.
- Nutritional deficiency, e.g. lack of methionine.

However, fatty change must persist for months, or even years, before the liver cells are irreversibly damaged and become incapable of a return to normal when the damaging agent is removed (59–60). Hydropic change is also a reversible process (61–64).

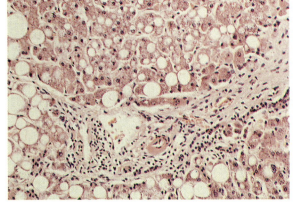

59 Cell vacuolation. Liver cells around the portal tract in the centre are bloated by large, round droplets of fat. The fat has been dissolved out of the tissue during the process of paraffin embedding. Droplets of fat often vary greatly in size. (*H and E × 10*)

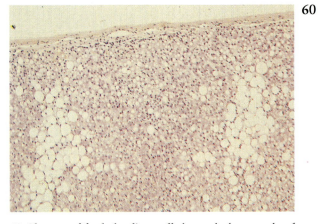

60 Clusters of fat laden liver cells beneath the capsule of the liver. A common post mortem finding, often related to terminal hypoxia. (*H and E × 20*)

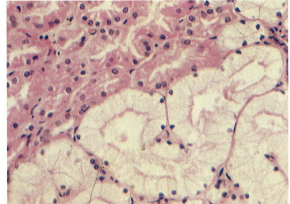

61 Patchy hydropic change in renal tubular cells. The cells at the lower part of the picture are swollen by water accumulation. (*H and E × 20*)

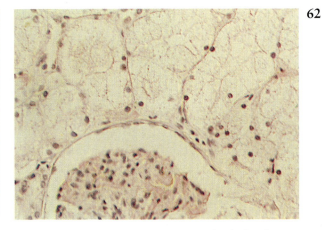

62 Extreme hydropic change in renal tubules from a patient treated with mannitol to promote diuresis. (*H and E × 20*)

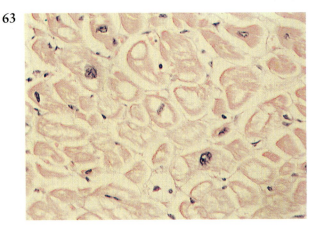

63 Hydropic change in subendocardial myocardial fibres caused by ischaemia (q.v.) due to coronary artery narrowing. (*H and E × 10*)

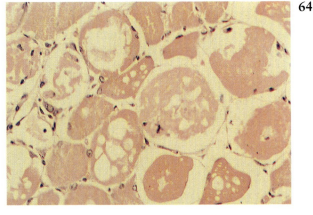

64 Hydropic change in ischaemic skeletal muscle fibres. From the tibialis anterior muscle, made ischaemic by a tight anterior compartment of the leg. (*H and E × 20*)

Accumulations in cells

A variety of substances may collect in cells and in supporting tissues in pathological states. Sometimes the accumulation is of physiological components in excess, for example, iron in the liver, copper in the liver and cornea, and glycogen in the liver. At other times the material that collects is an abnormal metabolite, or substance such as amyloid (q.v.). Diseases characterised by the appearance of such substances are sometimes called infiltrations. Examples of such materials are:

- Mucin.
- Lipid.
- Amyloid.
- Fibrinoid.
- Hyaline.
- Iron.
- Copper.
- Calcium.

Mucin is a loose term used to describe the appearance of mucopolysaccharides in the connective tissue, and to describe intracellular epithelial polysaccharides, as in colonic cells; both are mucosubstances. Mucin sometimes collects in the aortic wall, causing cystic gaps that weaken the wall and provoke aortic rupture: this is sometimes called aortic medionecrosis. There is a group of diseases called mucopolysaccharidoses characterised by a variety of these substances (mucosubstances) in various organs (65–68).

Lipid is found in reticuloendothelial cells of the liver, spleen, marrow and other organs. These rare disorders are called lipidoses, and different lipids collect in the various diseases.

Amyloid is an unusual extracellular fibrous protein, which accumulates in the connective tissues of the body. Immunochemical, x-ray diffraction and electron microscope studies have revealed the complexity of amyloid material. Amyloid material may be deposited with no obvious predisposing cause – so-called primary amyloidosis. Secondary amyloidosis follows chronic processes such as tuberculosis (q.v.), and there are other varieties that need not concern us here. Immunochemistry has shown secondary amyloidosis to be a protein called AA. Primary amyloid (AL) is the amino terminal of the light chain of immunoglobulins, or in a few cases, the whole light chain of a homogenous immunoglobulin. Other chemical types exist, and substances are present in the blood which may be precursors of amyloid (serum component (SAA) and plasma component (P)). Amyloid is red in H and E stained sections and is metachromatic with methyl violet, staining purple-red instead of the natural colour, violet. It also stains orange with Congo red, and shows apple green birefringence in polarised light. It stains a variety of colours with other dyes, but no staining method can recognise it specifically (70–77).

Fibrinoid and hyaline materials are eosinophilic, and resemble one another closely in histological appearance. Hyaline is a clear, glassy, amorphous eosinophilic material, that appears in droplets in cells (for example, in renal tubular cells where there is proteinuria) or in the connective tissues as in old scars. Hyalinisation of arteries is induced by radiation or hypertension, and hyaline arteries are often seen in the elderly (78–85). Fibrinoid is less glassy and more fragmented than hyaline, and is so named because it resembles fibrin in its staining appearances. Chemically, there are several kinds of fibrinoid, so it is not a homogenous entity (86–88).

Metals collect in tissues either because they are present in excess (for example, copper in Wilson's disease, ferric iron in haemochromatosis and transfusional siderosis of the liver, and calcium in hyperparathyroidism), or because they are deposited in dead or dying tissues (for example, calcium in old scars). These are more accumulations than infiltrations, and the material is often found within the cells (89–95).

Metastatic calcification is the deposition of calcium when the blood level is high; dystrophic calcification is the deposition of calcium into a dead or dying tissue (as in old tuberculous scars or in old arteries when the blood calcium level is normal).

65

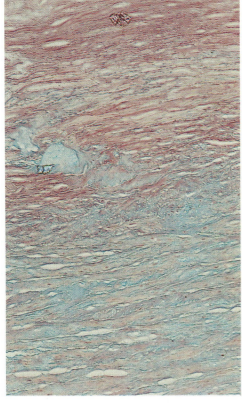

65 Accumulations in cells. Section of aortic wall showing focal accumulations of green mucosubstance scattered through the media. There is medial damage in the areas of mucosubstance accumulation, and the aorta may burst allowing blood to escape into body cavities or to track along the aorta under the adventitia (dissecting aneurysm). (*Alcian blue × 4*)

66

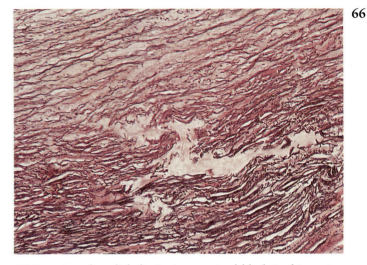

66 Fragmented medial elastic tissue stained black in this section of aortic wall. This leads to aortic rupture. (*Weigert's resorcin fuchsin ponceau S × 4*)

67

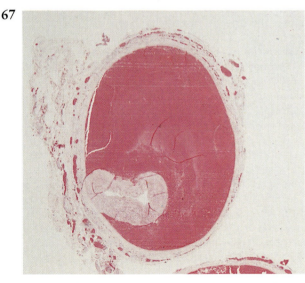

67 Blood has dissected the wall of this artery filling a space between media and adventitia. The inner part of the artery is seen bottom left. (*H and E*)

68

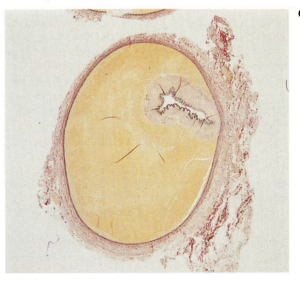

68 Accumulations. This stain shows elastic tissue black. It shows the site of dissection of the arterial wall, which occurs as blood tracks beneath the adventitia and along arterial branches that emerge from the aorta. (*Weigert's resorcin fuchsin ponceau S*)

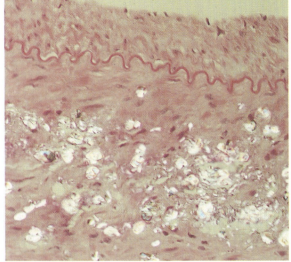

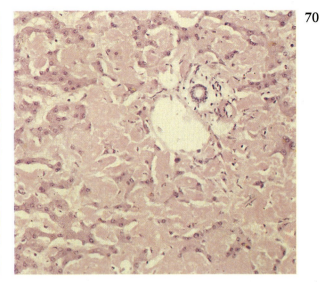

69 Accumulation of birefringent oxalate crystals in the arterial media from a case of oxalosis. This is an inborn error of metabolism in which there is over production of an oxalic acid compound by the liver. (*H and E and polariser × 4*)

70 Amyloid. Pink staining masses of amyloid separating and compressing liver cells in a portal area. (*H and E × 10*)

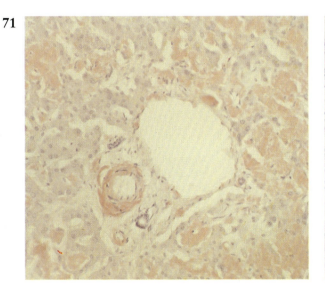

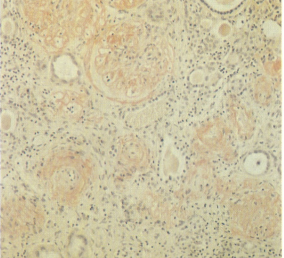

71 Amyloid in the liver, staining orange with Congo red. (*Congo red × 10*)

72 Amyloid. Low power view of kidney showing amyloid in glomerular tufts and in tubular basement membranes. (*Congo red × 4*)

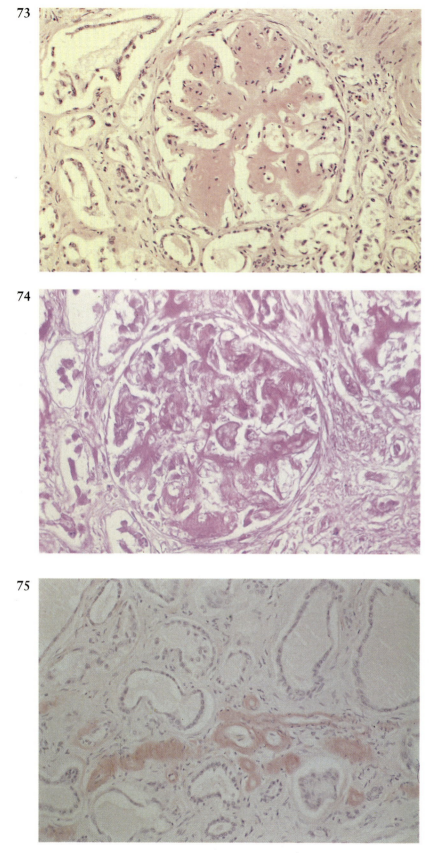

73 Glomerular tuft extensively infiltrated by amyloid. (*H and E × 10*)

74 Amyloid stains a purple colour with the dye methyl violet. (*Methyl violet × 10*)

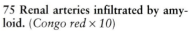

75 Renal arteries infiltrated by amyloid. (*Congo red × 10*)

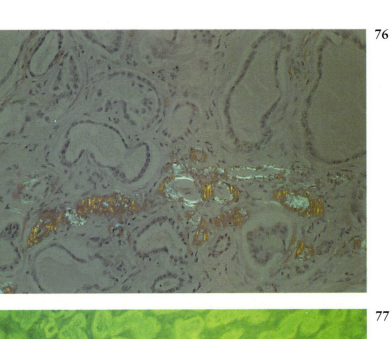

76 Amyloid. The same view as in **75** seen in polarised light. Amyloid exhibits a characteristic apple green birefringence. (*Congo red polariser ×10*)

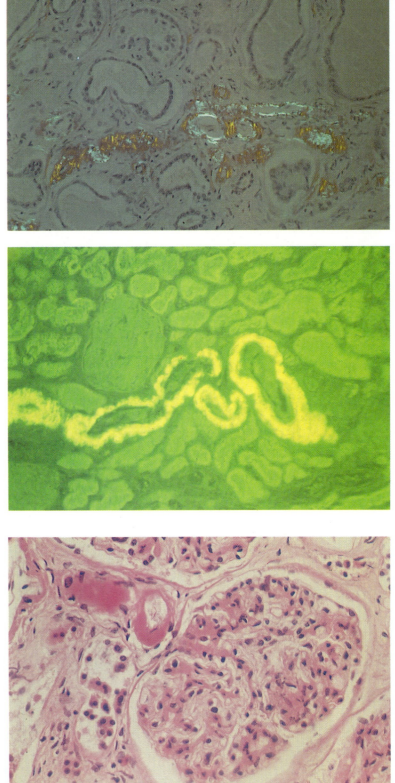

77 Renal vessels stained with thioflavin T and viewed in ultraviolet light. Thioflavin is a fluorochrome which binds to amyloid and fluoresces orange-yellow. (*Thioflavin T × 10*)

78 Hyaline. An afferent glomerular arteriole cut in two planes, showing replacement of the wall of the vessel by hyaline material. This is a common event in hypertensive heart disease. (*H and E × 20*)

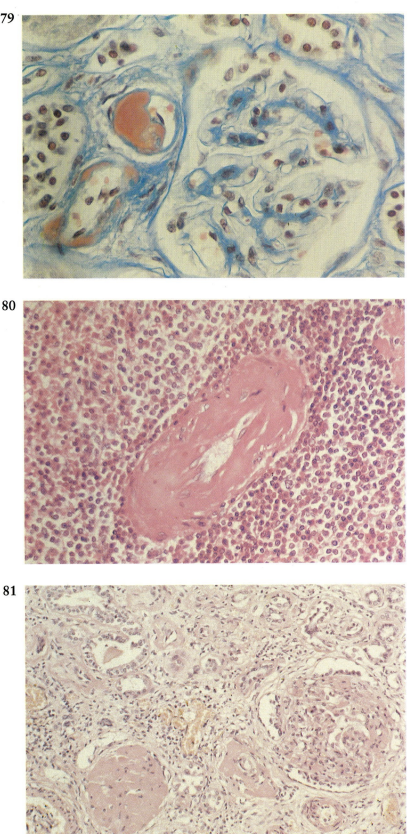

79 79 Pink, glassy hyaline material beneath the endothelium of an afferent glomerular arteriole. Stained by a trichrome method. (*McFarlane's modification of Mallory's trichrome stain × 20*)

80 Hyalinised arteriole in a Malpighian body in the spleen. This is a common finding starting in childhood. It has no relation to hypertensive heart disease (q.v.). (*H and E × 10*)

81 Hyaline. A glomerulus (bottom left) is totally replaced by hyaline collagen. A common finding in the kidney of the elderly. (*H and E × 4*)

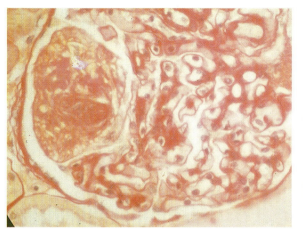

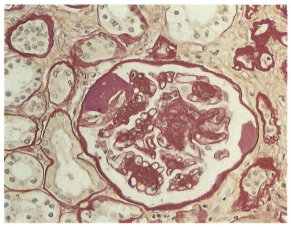

82 Hyaline thickening of glomerular tuft in a diabetic. The appearances are similar to those of amyloid. (*PAS × 20*)

83 Hyaline. Glomerular tuft from a diabetic. Hyaline deposits on the parietal layer of the glomerulus (known as capsular drops) are often seen in this condition. (*PAS × 10*)

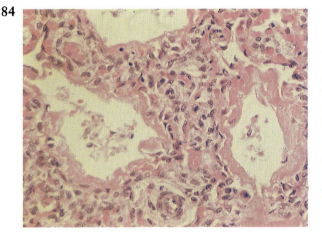

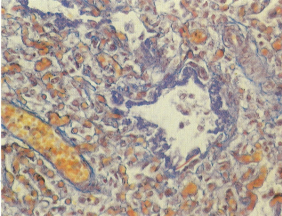

84 Hyaline. Pink staining hyaline membranes from a child with respiratory distress syndrome, caused by failure to produce adequate surfactant in the premature child. The membranes line the alveoli. (*H and E × 20*)

85 Hyaline. It is often difficult to distinguish hyaline material from fibrin and fibrinoid. Trichrome stains usually colour fibrin and fibrinoid red, but hyaline is not stained. Here the hyaline membranes stain blue. (*McFarlane's modification of Mallory's trichrome stain × 20*)

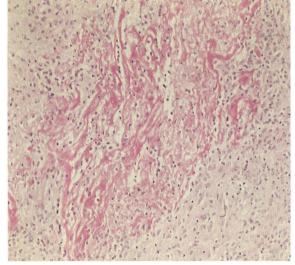

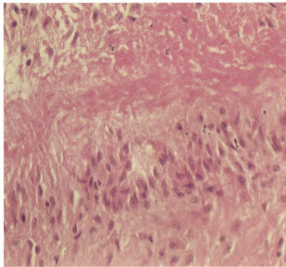

86 Fibrinoid material (top left) on the base of a chronic peptic ulcer in the stomach. (*H and E × 4*)

87 Fibrinoid (above) in a rheumatoid granuloma. The fibrinoid material is bordered by a palisade of histiocytes. (*H and E × 20*)

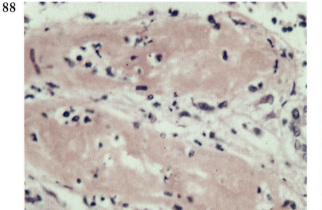

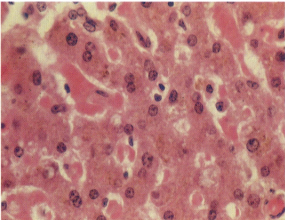

88 Fibrinoid necrosis in the renal vessels of a patient with malignant hypertension. The vessel wall is replaced by fibrinoid material and contains fragments of necrotic cells. (*H and E × 20*)

89 Iron. Abundant brown granules of iron in the liver of a patient who had received many blood transfusions. (*H and E × 20*)

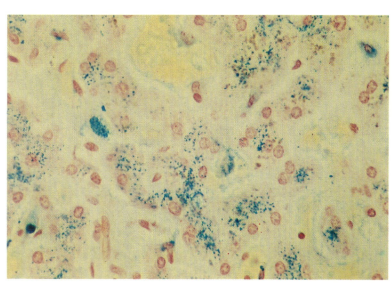

90 Iron. Special stains for ferric iron show blue granules of iron in liver and Kupffer cells. (*Perls' × 20*)

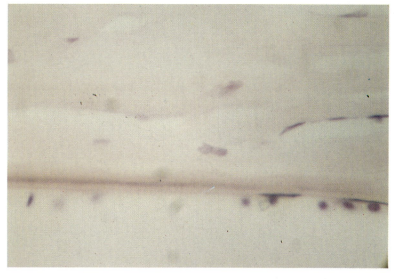

91 Copper. A thin black line of copper in the corneal Descemet's membrane. From a case of Wilson's disease, where excess copper is deposited in many tissues including the eye. (*Rubeanic acid × 40*)

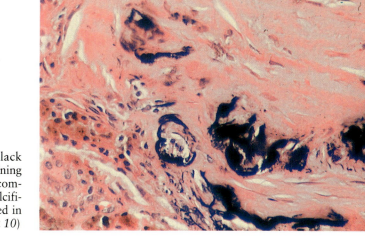

92 Dystrophic calcification. Black deposits of calcium in pink staining old scar tissue. This is not uncommon, and is called dystrophic calcification where calcium is deposited in old damaged tissues. (*H and E × 10*)

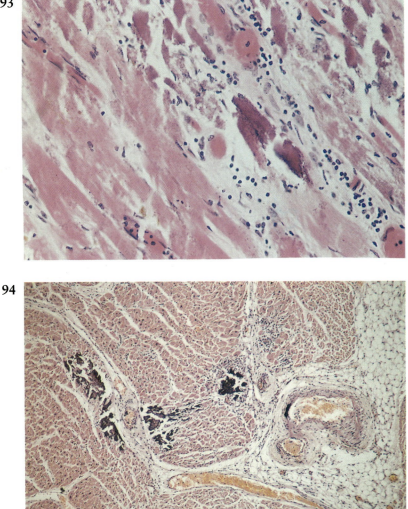

93 Dystrophic calcification in dead myocardial fibres in a cardiac infarct (q.v.). The calcium deposits are purple-black. (*H and E × 10*)

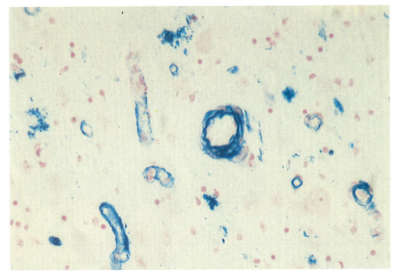

94 Metastatic calcification in undamaged heart muscle. This is caused by a raised blood level of calcium as in hyperparathyroidism. (*H and E × 2*)

95 Iron is sometimes deposited in cerebral infarcts (q.v.) together with calcium. This shows iron encrusted vessels in a region of dead (necrotic) brain tissue. (*Perls' × 20*)

Autolysis

This is an irrevocable affair. Hydrolytic enzymes are released from cells in which the lysosomal membranes have broken down, and then the cell virtually digests itself. Autolysis occurs post mortem as a usual event in the breakdown of the body. Before death, it is the late result of cell injury. It is often difficult to distinguish post mortem from ante mortem autolysis, but nuclear changes tend to be severe if the cell has been injured during life (**96, 97**).

Autolysis is more conspicuous in some organs than others. It is commonly seen after death in the gut and other glandular organs, such as the pancreas, kidneys and suprarenals.

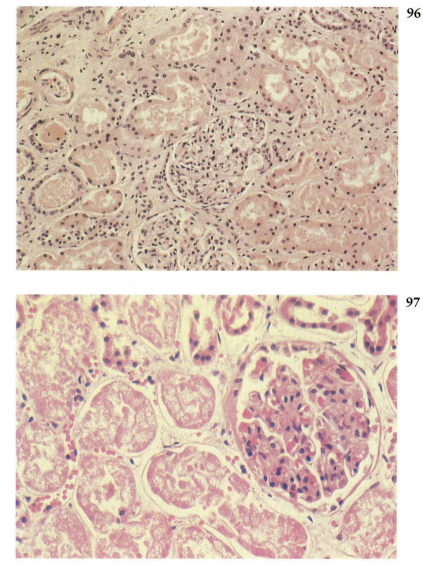

96

96 Autolysis. Kidney showing autolytic breakdown of tubular epithelial cells. It is also the basis of the change called cloudy swelling which has been described earlier. (*H and E × 10*)

97

97 Advanced severe autolysis of renal tubular cells. Glomerulus is well preserved. (*H and E × 10*)

Necrosis

This means death of a cell or tissue. Necrotic changes are made up of cytoplasmic alterations (already described) and the nuclear changes of:

- *Pyknosis,* which is intense nuclear shrinkage, often seen in severe damage, e.g. burning of a tissue (98).
- *Karyorrhexis,* here the nucleus breaks into fragments. Such fragments are commonly seen in reactive centres in lymph nodes.
- *Karyolysis,* where the nucleus swells and lyses (99, 100).
- *Apoptosis,* which means dropping off, and applies to the death of single cells or small groups of cells. It occurs in many conditions, notably to liver cells in viral hepatitis (101).

So far we have described the microscopical appearances of necrosis, but necrotic tissue is also seen macroscopically and presents various appearances:

- *Coagulative* necrosis, where the tissue retains its shape but is dead, e.g. a renal or cardiac infarct (q.v.) (108).
- *Liquefactive* necrosis, as in the brain, where the dead tissue liquefies and forms a cyst (109).
- *Caseous* necrosis, caused by *M. tuberculosis.* The consistency is soft and cheesy due to lipid from the organism (110).
- *Gaseous* necrosis (gas gangrene), where bacteria (Clostridia) kill muscle and ferment the glycogen to produce gas bubbles (107).
- *Gummatous* necrosis, or rubbery necrosis, where fibrous tissue replacement keeps pace with cell destruction, as in syphilis.
- *Fat* necrosis, where omental and other fat becomes necrotic and opaque, due to the liberation of fatty acids by lipases from a diseased pancreas (pancreatitis) (111).

98

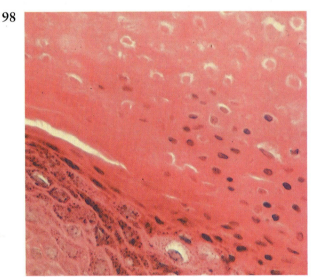

98 Pyknosis in normal skin. Nuclei of cells of the stratum granulosum (bottom left) shrink as they move to the surface. The nuclei then lose their haematoxophilia (top right), and the keratin flakes that come off the skin surface are normally anuclear. (*H and E × 20*)

99

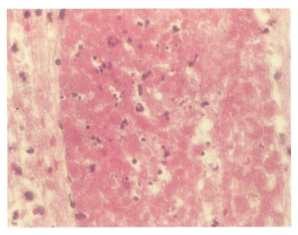

99 Necrotic tissue showing fragmentation and shrinkage of nuclei, and coagulation and loss of outlines of cell cytoplasm. A typical appearance of necrosis. (*H and E × 40*)

100 Karyolysis. An area of necrosis showing vacuolate lysed cells (karyolysis) top right. (*H and E × 20*)

101 Apoptosis. A group of liver cells in the centre showing shrunken eosinophilic cytoplasm and pyknotic nuclei. This individual cell death is apoptosis. (*H and E × 20*)

102 Necrosis. Liver showing a portal tract in the centre. Liver cells in the mid and central areas of the lobule are necrotic. (*H and E × 4*)

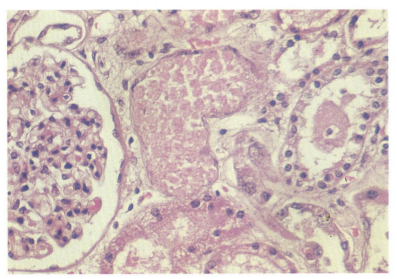

103 Necrosis. A renal tubule in the centre shows total epithelial necrosis. (× 10)

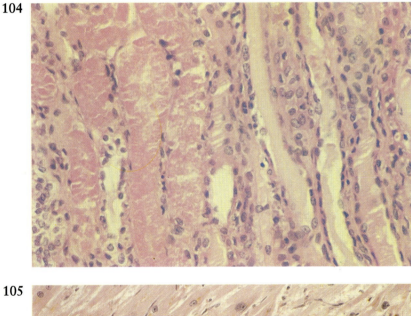

104 Necrotic renal tubules on the left seen in longitudinal section. Those on the right are moderately well preserved. (*H and E × 10*)

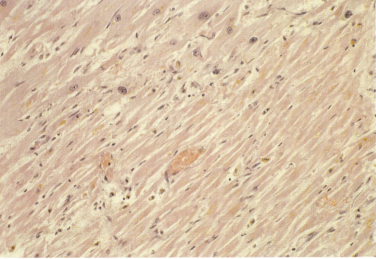

105 Necrotic cardiac muscle (bottom right). Nuclear staining has been lost in the dead fibres. (*H and E × 4*)

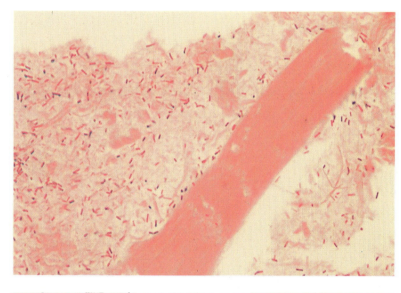

106 Necrotic fragmented skeletal muscle. The chains and bunches of nuclei are the result of sarcolemmal proliferation, in an attempt to repair the damage. (*H and E × 20*)

107 Anucleate necrotic skeletal muscle. The surrounding tissue contains many black rod-shaped bacilli (Clostridia) which are the causative organisms of gas gangrene. (*Gram stain × 40*)

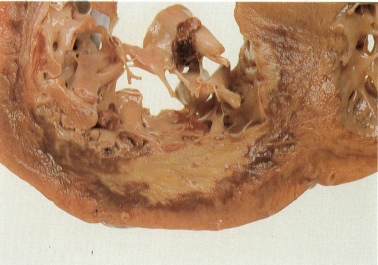

108 Coagulative necrosis. A slice of left ventricle showing a yellow area of coagulative necrosis in the wall bordered by a purple rim. This is an inflammatory response (q.v.) to the dead heart muscle.

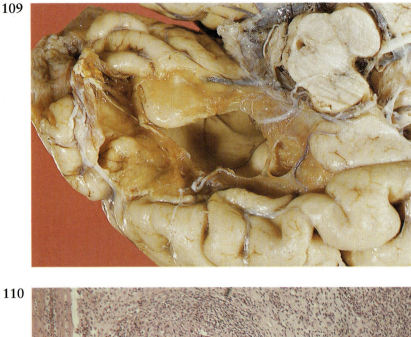

109 Liquefactive necrosis. A view of the inferior aspect of the left occipital pole of the brain, showing an area of liquefactive necrosis. The dead brain tissue has been absorbed, leaving a cavity. The cavity is stained brown by haemosiderin derived from broken down red blood cells.

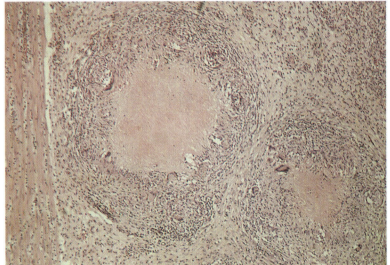

110 Pink caseous necrosis at the centre of tuberculous follicles (q.v.). The central necrotic area is bordered by mononuclear cells and giant cells. (*H and E × 2*)

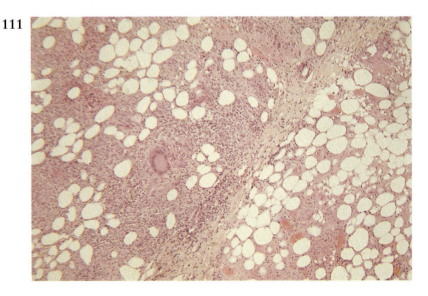

111 Necrotic fat (bottom right), the cells have lost their nuclear staining. There is an inflammatory reaction (q.v.) containing a giant cell (q.v.) in the adjacent fatty tissue. This is a response to the fat necrosis. (*H and E × 4*)

5 Causes of cellular damage

We do not know the causes of the two main fatal diseases of the Western world, *viz.* obliterative arterial disease (q.v.) and neoplasia ('cancer') (q.v.). More is known of infectious agents which, although they have been suppressed by hygienic measures and antibiotic drugs in the West, still represent the main cause of illness and death worldwide.

Animate agents

Viruses, rickettsiae, mycoplasmas

This covers organisms which vary greatly in size. At one end of the scale are the obligate intracellular agents like viruses and rickettsiae, and at the other are large tapeworms occupying much of the small gut.

Viral diseases are common and sometimes, like influenza, notorious. Many viruses produce inclusion bodies in the cells they infect. The appearances of the inclusion and its position (whether in the nucleus or cytoplasm or both) gives a clue to the nature of the infection. For example, the cytomegalovirus of the herpes group enlarges the nucleus with its inclusion, producing an 'owl's eye' appearance (**112–117**).

Rickettsiae are intracellular, arthropod-borne organisms. Ornithosis, trachoma and cat scratch disease were once thought to be viral in origin. However, it is now known that ornithosis and trachoma are due to *Chlamydia*, and cat scratch disease is thought to be of bacterial origin (**118, 119**).

Mycoplasmas resemble the L (Lister) forms of bacteria. They are ubiquitous and are associated with a variety of diseases of man and animals. Mycoplasmal pneumonia is so common in the pig as to be almost a usual finding at slaughter. The lesions are characteristic, but the organism (like the rickettsiae) is difficult to find in sections (**120**).

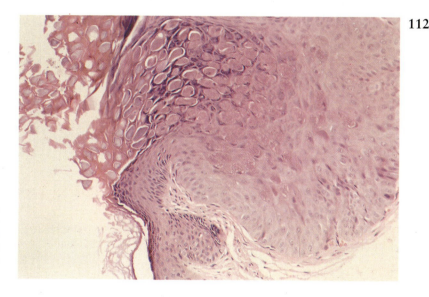

112

112 Virus. Molluscum contagiosum, a virus induced lesion of the skin. The normal epidermis is below, and the lesion is in the upper part of the section. Note the large, pink viral inclusion bodies. (*H and E × 10*)

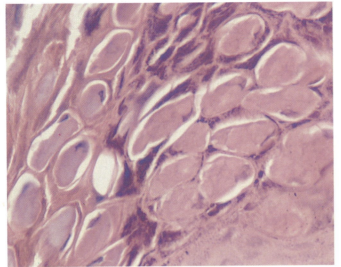

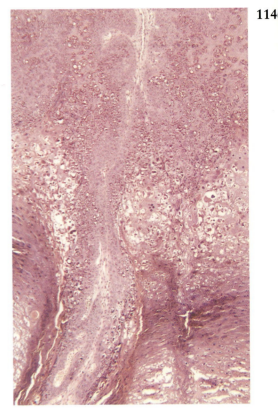

113 Molluscum contagiosum, high power view showing pink inclusion bodies. (*H and E × 40*)

114 Common wart of skin. The epidermis is totally disorganised and contains many inclusion bodies. (*H and E × 4*)

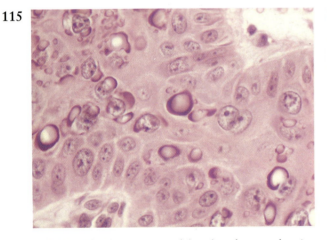

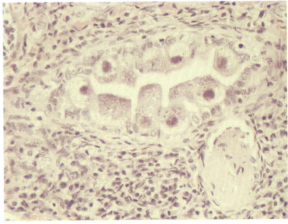

115 Wart. High power view of the edge of a wart showing large purple inclusions in the epithelial cells. (*H and E × 40*)

116 Cytomegalovirus. Renal tubule from a kidney homograft (q.v.) showing cytomegalovirus inclusions in the epithelium. (*H and E × 20*)

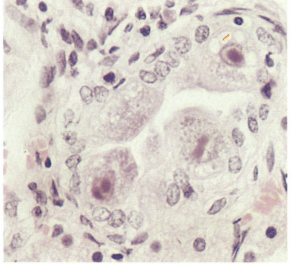

117 Inclusions of cytomegalovirus in renal tubular cells showing typical 'owl's eye' appearance. This virus is a common opportunistic invader of transplanted organs. (*H and E × 40*)

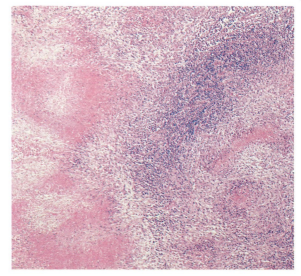

118 Cat scratch disease. Bands of pink necrosis in a lymph node from a case of cat scratch fever. The agent was classed as a rickettsia, but is now thought to be a bacterium, transmitted by a scratch of a cat. The organism reaches a local lymph node where it produces the lesion. (*H and E × 2*)

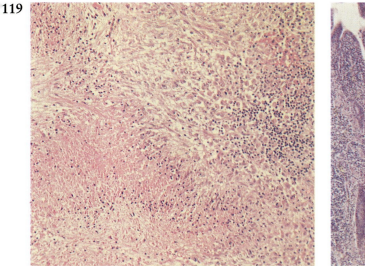

119 Cat scratch disease. A higher power view of a lymph node from cat scratch disease. The lesion is a granuloma (q.v.), showing an area of necrosis bordered by macrophages and lymphocytes. (*H and E × 10*)

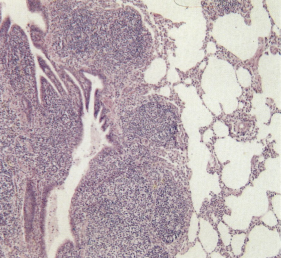

120 Mycoplasmal pneumonia. Section of lung showing numerous lymphoid follicles around a bronchiole. This is a typical picture of the late stage of mycoplasmal pneumonia. (*H and E × 4*)

Bacteria and fungi

Bacteria can often be seen in sections of diseased tissues stained by Gram's method. Some appear as black dots or clumps. They can be readily distinguished from coal dust or other artefacts by their regular shape and size. Other bacteria are recognised by different staining methods. For example, carbol fuchsin in the Ziehl Neelsen method is used to identify mycobacteria. Silver methods are needed to outline spirochaetes, such as the causative organism of syphilis (**121–134**).

Fungi are often difficult to see as they stain weakly basophilic with H and E. However, a periodic acid-Schiff (PAS) or other special stain, such as a silver method, reveals them clearly. It is important to think of a possible fungal cause when faced with a section of an obscure chronic inflammation. A periodic acid-Schiff or Grocott silver stain will rapidly reveal the solution to the problem. Fungi, especially Candida and Aspergillus, are frequent invaders of transplanted organs (**135–146**).

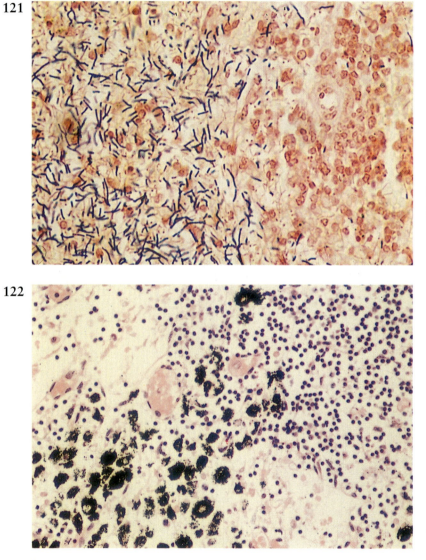

121 **121 *Bacillus anthracis.*** A section of lymph node draining a skin lesion in a butcher who was infected from handling contaminated meat. The organisms are abundant Gram-positive *Bacillus anthracis* rods of even width. (*Gram stain × 40*)

122 **122 Coal dust** in the lung. Dust particles are of variable size, often occur in clumps and can easily be distinguished from microorganisms. (*H and E × 20*)

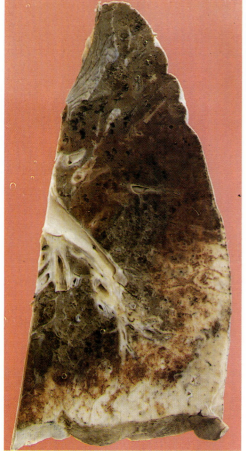

123 Staphylococcal pneumonia. Slice of lung showing dark areas of haemorrhage. This is an acute staphylococcal pneumonia. The organism produces toxins that damage vascular endothelium and give rise to the haemorrhagic pneumonia.

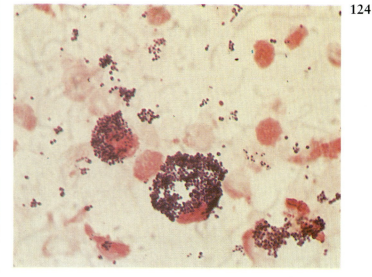

124 Staphylococcal pneumonia. A smear of pus (q.v.) from the trachea of the lung shown in **123**. Gram-positive cocci are present free and in phagocytes which have pink nuclei. (*Gram stain × 40*)

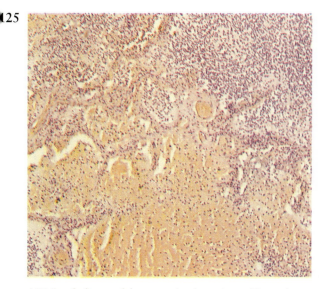

125 Staphylococcal pneumonia. A section of lung showing polymorphonuclear leucocytes in some alveoli (top), and haemorrhage into the alveoli (below). (*H and E × 4*)

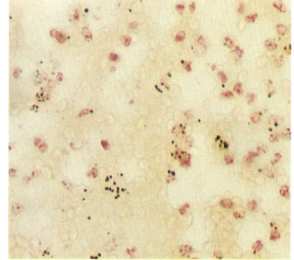

126 Staphylococcal pneumonia. Gram stain of the lung shown in **125**, showing numerous Gram-positive, black cocci and leucocytes in the alveoli. (*Gram stain × 40*)

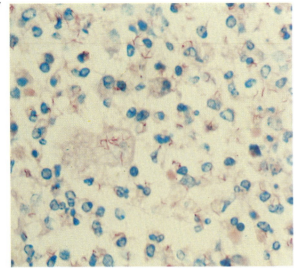

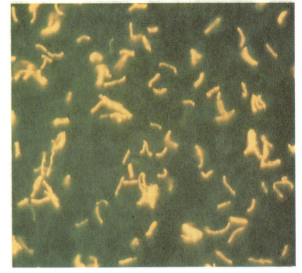

127 *Mycobacterium tuberculosis* in a lymph node. The organism stains red with carbol fuchsin, and resists decolorisation with acid and alcohol. It is said to be acid alcohol fast. In the centre a macrophage contains bacilli. (*Ziehl Neelsen × 40*)

128 Acid alcohol fast bacilli are often sparse in lesions, but their presence is diagnostic of tuberculosis. They can be sought by staining with the fluorochrome auramine, and then searching the section under ultraviolet light when they fluoresce orange. (*Auramine × 100*)

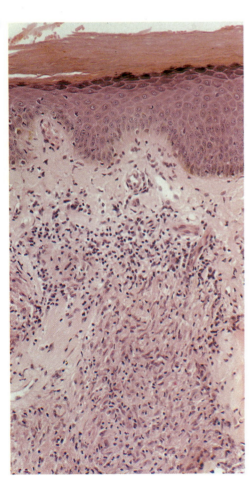

129 Leprosy. Section of skin from a case of leprosy. The lesion is a granuloma (q.v.) composed largely of macrophages, so-called 'lepra cells' (below). (*H and E × 10*)

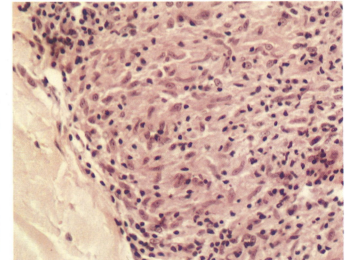

130 Leprosy. Higher power view of the granuloma of cutaneous leprosy. The macrophages are spindle-shaped and referred to as epithelioid cells. A sprinkling of lymphocytes is present. (*H and E × 20*)

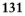

131

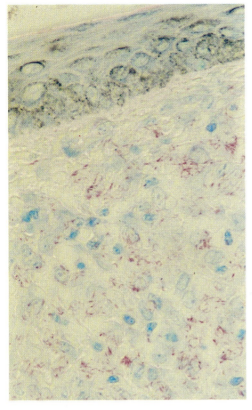

131 *M. leprae.* Epidermis (above) showing many melanocytes. The lesion in the dermis shows numerous red staining rods which are the bacilli of *Mycobacterium leprae.* They often occur in clumps and have hazy outlines particularly after treatment of the patient with dapsone. (*Modified Ziehl Neelsen × 40*)

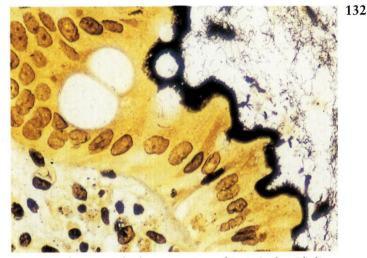

132

132 Spirochaetes. A high power view of intestinal epithelium showing a dense black layer of spirochaetes on the surface. Individual organisms can be seen on the right of the picture. (*Levaditi silver method × 40*)

133

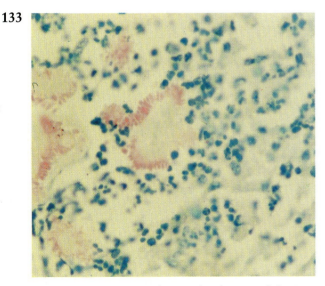

133 Actinomycosis is a bacterial infection of the jaw, gut and liver, caused by an organism which is intermediate between bacteria and fungi. In sections it stains as acid fast rods in a 'sun ray' appearance, hence its name. The section shows red rods surrounded by leucocytes. (*Ziehl Neelsen × 40*)

134

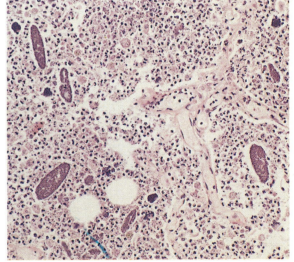

134 Bacterial proliferation continues in the body after death. This shows oval, dark clumps of organisms embedded in leucocytes. It is likely that few organisms were present originally, and these clumps represent post mortem proliferation. (*H and E × 10*)

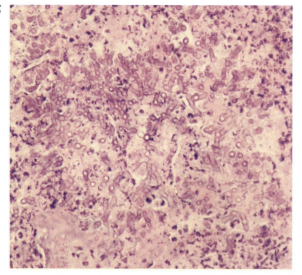

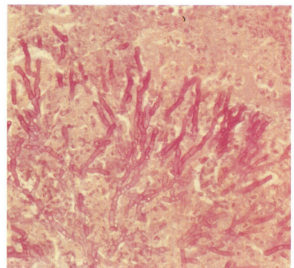

135 Aspergillary hyphae in purulent exudate from the lung of a patient with a kidney transplant. (*H and E × 20*)

136 Hyphae of *Aspergillus fumigatus* stained magenta by the periodic acid-Schiff method. The hyphae are broad branched and segmented. (*PAS × 20*)

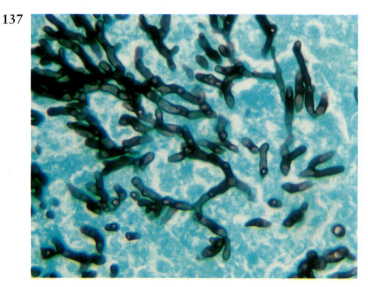

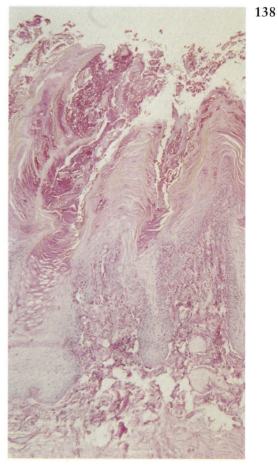

137 Grocott's silver method is a useful stain for identifying fungi. It stains the hyphae black. (*Grocott silver × 40*)

138 *Candida albicans*. Section of tongue showing papillae covered by magenta staining fungus. This is *Candida albicans* which is both a yeast and filamentous fungus. (*PAS × 4*)

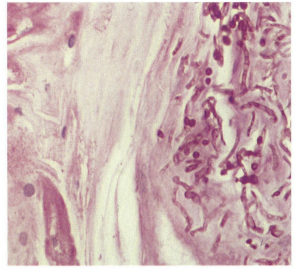

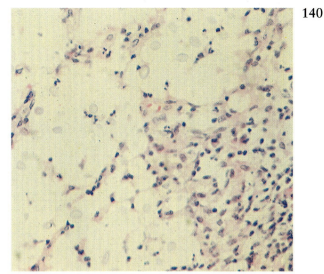

139 *Candida albicans.* High power view of the tongue showing fungus to the right. The filaments and rounded yeast forms of *Candida albicans* are visible. (*PAS × 40*)

140 *Cryptococcus neoformans.* Section of lung from a cryptococcal infection. *Cryptococcus neoformans* is a yeast like Candida, but it also has a capsule. It may be difficult to see in H and E sections, and is barely visible as pale grey bodies in this section. (*H and E × 20*)

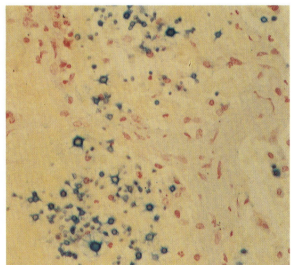

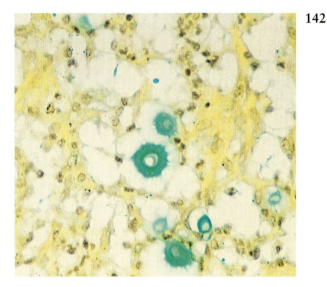

141 Alcian blue. Special stains, such as alcian blue, stain the capsule and make the organism readily visible. (*Alcian blue × 20*)

142 Cryptococcus. A higher power view to show the cell wall and capsule of the cryptococcus. (*Alcian blue × 40*)

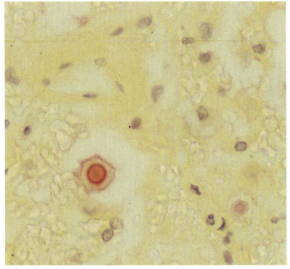

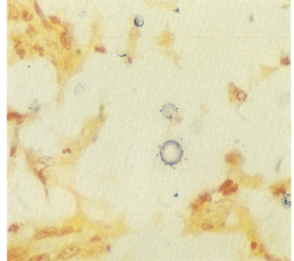

143 The cryptococcal capsule also stains with the dye mucicarmine. Here the periphery of the capsule is pink and the body of the organism is red. (*Mucicarmine × 40*)

144 The cell wall of the cryptococcus is Gram-positive. (*Gram stain × 40*)

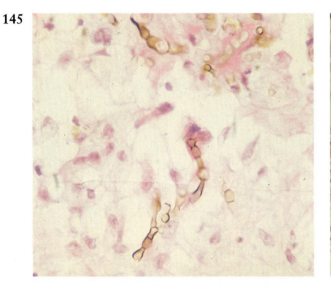

145 Forisecaea. Brown flask-shaped fragments of a fungus from a case of chromoblastomycosis. The pigmented organism *Forisecaea pedrosoi* causes large skin lesions in rural areas of the Caribbean. Fungal fragments may be sparse in the lesions. (*H and E × 40*)

146 Forisecaea. A giant celled granuloma caused by Forisecaea species. The fungal elements are sparse in the giant cells. In any unexplained granuloma fungi should be sought by the use of special stains. (*H and E × 20*)

Protozoa

Malaria is a protozoal disorder that causes much disease worldwide. However, this and other protozoal disorders are uncommon in Western temperate countries. A recent small increase in protozoal infections has occurred in Britain, because of the use of immunosuppressive agents to enable transplanted organs to survive in a foreign host. These drugs, like azothioprine, damp down the response to foreign proteins and also to most microorganisms, including cytomegalovirus, fungi and protozoa. Some of the latter are Sporozoa, such as *Toxoplasma gondii* and *Pneumocystis carinii*, that may be found in abundance in the lungs and other tissues of people dying after organ transplantation (147–154).

147

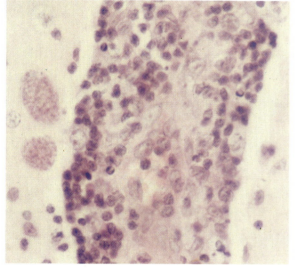

148

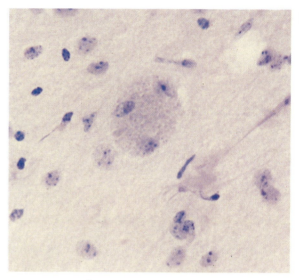

147 *Toxoplasma gondii*. Two cysts of the protozoan *Toxoplasma gondii* alongside a blood vessel in the brain, and surrounded by lymphoid plasma cells. (*H and E × 40*)

148 Toxoplasmosis. A cyst in the brain, containing the bow-shaped organisms of toxoplasmosis. (*H and E × 40*)

149

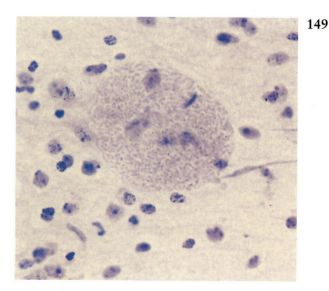

149 *Toxoplasma gondii* cyst showing the details of the organism. (*H and E × 80*)

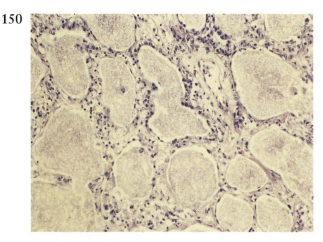

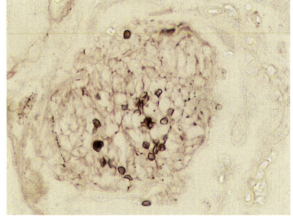

150 *Pneumocystis carinii.* A low power view of a section of lung from a child with treated leukaemia (q.v.). The alveoli contain amorphous pink material. These are masses of the trophozoites of *Pneumocystis carinii*, a common opportunistic organism in immunodepleted subjects. Note the epithelialisation of the alveoli. (*H and E × 10*)

151 The trophozoites of Pneumocystis are often difficult to find in H and E sections, but they can be shown up easily by using the Grocott silver stain. Here they appear as black objects which are occasionally typically cup-shaped. (*Grocott stain × 40*)

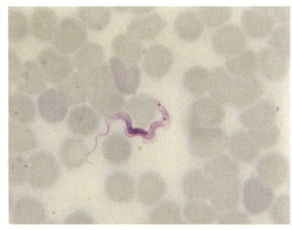

152 Trypanosoma. Some protozoa have flagella and swim in the bloodstream, and then settle in various organs, such as the heart and colon, to produce disease. This is a blood film showing a flagellate Trypanosoma. The flagellum is to the left. (*Leishman stain × 100*)

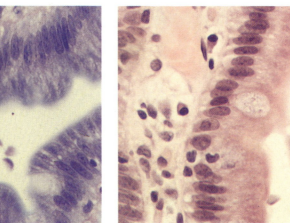

153 Giardia. Some flagellate protozoa such as *Giardia lamblia* live in the gut. They can often be shown better by Giemsa stain. They can be seen here in the space between the gut epithelial cells. (*Giemsa × 40*)

154 Giardia are flagellates with a sucker. They attach themselves to the surface of gut epithelial cells, as shown here. They cause malabsorbtion of food materials when present in the small bowel. (*H and E × 40*)

Metazoa

Medical practitioners are, in general, unaware of the possibility of fungal, protozoal and metazoal infections, yet all three can cause serious diseases. Metazoa include a diverse range of parasites, many of them helminths (worms). Some, like tapeworms and pinworms (Cestoda and Nematoda), are relatively trivial infections. Others, like the liver flukes (Trematoda), cause widespread diseases worldwide with high morbidity rates.

Particularly serious are the migrating larvae of certain ascarid worms (*Toxocara canis* and *T. cati*). These worms, present in the faeces of dogs and cats, are swallowed by children, and the larvae migrate through the tissues (visceral larva migrans). Some of them finish up in the eye, and cause a reaction that leads to blindness. In Britain, toxocariasis is one of the most common causes of blindness in children (**155–160**).

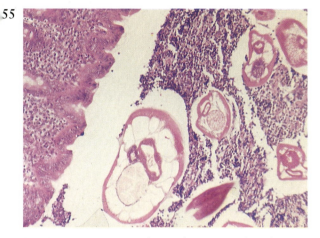

155 Metazoa. Section of vermiform appendix, showing transverse section of the common threadworm or pinworm of children, mingled with lymphocytes in the lumen of the appendix. (*H and E × 4*)

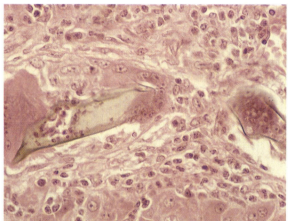

156 *Schistosoma mansoni* eggs in a portal tract in the liver. The egg on the left has a lateral pointed spine, characteristic of this trematode. Giant cells have mounted a reaction against the egg. (*H and E × 20*)

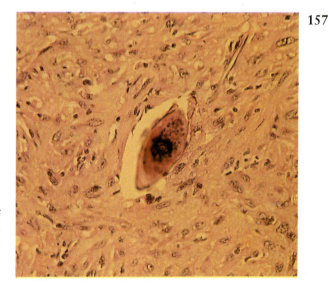

157 An egg of *Schistosoma haematobium* in the wall of the urinary bladder, surrounded by a dense chronic inflammatory response (q.v.). Persistent irritation by this worm leads to bladder ulceration and ultimately to bladder cancer. (*H and E × 20*)

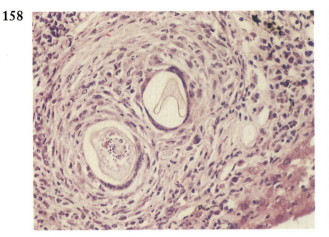

158 Schistosoma. Another example of the dense fibrocellular response to the eggs of schistosomas. (*H and E × 20*)

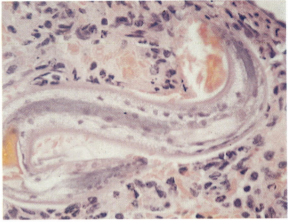

159 Migrating larva of *Toxocara canis* in the lung. Such larvae are unable to escape from the circulation into the lung and gut, and may migrate to the eye causing blindness. (*H and E × 20*)

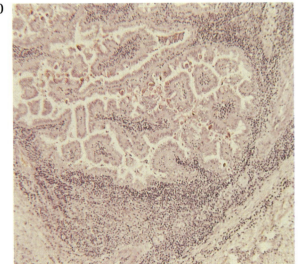

160 Trematode. Papillary proliferation of bile duct epithelium that can lead to carcinoma (q.v.). This is produced by trematode worms in the biliary tree. (*H and E × 4*)

Inanimate agents

The environment is bristling with potentially dangerous agents of all kinds: radiations, dusts and smokes, preservatives in food, drugs and poisons. Some people are more exposed than others, for example, workers with asbestos, silica, cotton dust and so on are likely to develop disease as a result of inhalation of these agents. Sections of diseased tissues sometimes reveal the cause, for example, iron-coated asbestos particles may be seen in a section of fibrotic lung, but often the cause is not apparent (**161, 162**).

Radiation affects tissues either by stimulating cell division or, if the dose is large enough, by killing cells. It also acts more subtly by causing a progressive swelling of arterial walls, leading to vascular occlusion and ischaemia. Radiations act at a molecular level, either by scoring 'hits' on nuclear DNA, or by producing toxic ionic products of water that damage cells (**163–167**).

Poison is a general term for a wide range of agents. Some act subtly by interfering with the intermediary metabolism (for example, carbon monoxide or fluoracetate), while others are crude corrosive agents, like acids and alkalis, that destroy cells. Often the poisons tend to act on specific cells, like the diphtheria toxin on certain neurons, the aflatoxin (from *Aspergillus flavus*) on the liver, strychnine on the anterior spinal cord neurons, and so on.

Vascular tissues seem to be especially prone to a number of toxic agents. One of the more interesting groups of these are the alkaloids from the plants that form the basis of Jamaican bush tea. These substances cause intimal proliferation of veins and probably endocardial thickening in the heart. The venous intimal proliferation is seen par-ticularly in the liver, where vessels throughout the organ become occluded. This is veno-occlusive disease.

Dry or wet heat will coagulate tissue and, if intense enough, char it and reduce it to a carbon residue. Electrical injury produces damage by both heat and electrolysis, so an electrical burn shows charring and blistering (**168**). A general rise of body temperature, due to failure of temperature control, can lead to the death of neurons in the brain and the tearing of skeletal muscle by hypercontraction. This occurs during anaesthesia in a few individuals sensitive to succinylcholine and other agents (**169**).

161

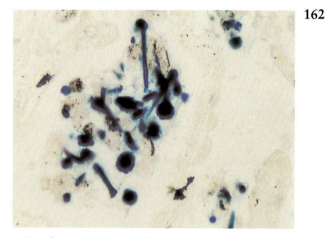

161 Asbestos fibres. Brown staining particles of asbestos fibres in alveoli. The alveolar walls are thickened by pink fibrous tissue, and coal dust is present (bottom left). (*H and E × 20*)

162

162 Asbestos particles of characteristic shape. They stain blue because they are coated with ferric iron. (*Perls' stain × 40*)

163

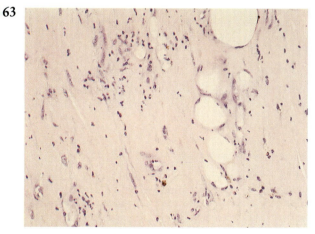

163 Irradiation. Section of the breast after previous irradiation, showing dense pink fibrous tissue enclosing a few adipose tissue cells. Occasional plump fibroblasts are present. (*H and E × 10*)

164

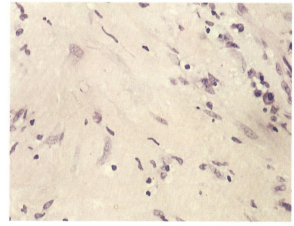

164 Irradiation. Scattered plump fibroblasts and occasional plasma cells in dense fibrous tissue following irradiation. (*H and E × 20*)

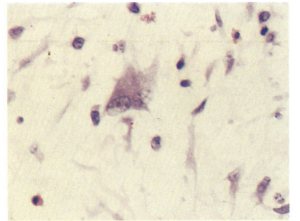

165 Irradiation. Detail of the large angular fibroblasts that appear after irradiation of a tissue by x-rays. (*H and E × 40*)

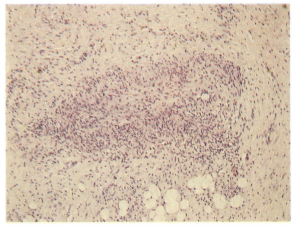

166 Irradiation. Dense, chronically inflamed fibrous tissue enclosing an artery (centre), the lumen of which has been obliterated by cellular proliferation. Such vascular changes follow irradiation and make the tissue avascular. Irradiated tissues are consequently susceptible to damage, and do not heal well after injury. (*H and E × 10*)

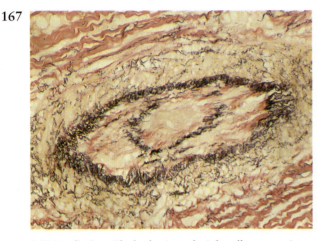

167 Irradiation. Black elastic and pink collagenous tissue proliferation in an irradiated artery in the treatment of breast cancer. (*Weigert's resorcin fuchsin ponceau S × 10*)

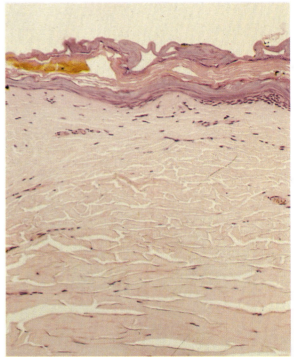

168 Skin from a burn caused by lightning. The surface epithelium has coagulated and lost its cell detail, and the cell nuclei are characteristically elongated. The underlying dermis shows spaces due to gas formation by electrolysis. (*H and E × 10*)

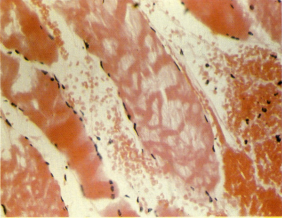

169 Hyperthermia. Skeletal muscle from a young girl who died of malignant hyperthermia following the administration of an anaesthetic to remove her appendix. The excessive contracture of muscle has led to tearing and fragmentation of the fibres. (*H and E × 20*)

6 Responses to cellular damage

This is probably the most important chapter in this book, for it illustrates the basic responses of living things when they are injured, whatever the injurious agent may be.

The reactions are local ones at or near the portal entry of the agent, and general reactions that may occur throughout the body; these come into play when the disease-producing stimulus is strong enough to elicit the general reaction. The general reaction is often a leucocytosis, which is a rise in blood polymorphonuclear leucocytes produced by the bone marrow.

If a staphylococcus enters a hair follicle on the skin surface it provokes an inflammation in the skin that may prevent the organism from spreading. If the organism succeeds in spreading it does so by the lymphatics to the regional lymph nodes, where the phagocytic cells of the reticulo-endothelial system multiply. This mechanism may also fail so that the organisms enter the bloodstream, causing a general response composed of fever, a rise in the white blood count (leucocytosis), and a steady rise in the level of antibody globulins derived from lymphoid cells. The role of fever and its cause is still obscure. Leucocytosis might be envisaged as providing more phagocytic cells for the ingestion and destruction of the organism. Antibodies, when they appear, are opsonic; that is they promote phagocytosis as well as other actions (**170–177**).

If all fails then septicaemia results: the bacteria multiply in the bloodstream and the host may die. Bacteraemia is a state where bacteria are present in the blood, but their growth is arrested by the suppressant effect of antibodies. Pyaemia is a grave event where the dividing bacteria and particles of necrotic material gain entry to the blood, usually via a vein in the wall of a necrotic zone of tissue. Here, then, are two serious effects: toxin production by bacteria, and ischaemia caused by vascular blockage by necrotic debris.

Phagocytes are microphages (polymorphonuclear neutrophils) and macrophages (variously called monocytes, histiocytes, littoral cells, Kupffer cells, etc). Antibodies aid their action, forming the most potent deterrent in bacterial infections.

Eosinophil leucocytes sometimes appear in large numbers, especially in helminth infections and in allergic disorders. They are phagocytic and produce histaminase. This enzyme destroys histamine derived from mast cells, which causes blood vessels to dilate in inflammation and in allergic reactions (q.v.).

Thrombocytosis is a rise in the platelet count of the blood. This is a delayed response, taking a few days to develop, and often follows extensive trauma or splenectomy. It may be envisaged as a protective mechanism to encourage thrombosis in blood vessels (q.v.), thereby preventing bleeding that might occur after tissue damage.

Phagocytosis

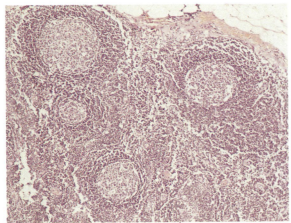

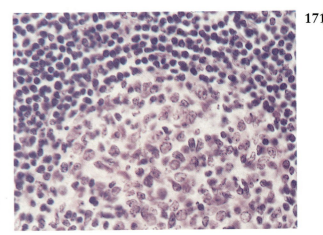

170 Phagocytosis. Germinal, reactive centres in the cortex of a lymph node. These are a source of B lymphocytes that produce immunoglobulins. (*H and E × 4*)

171 Phagocytosis. High power view of a reactive centre in a lymph node. Also called a germinal centre or follicle. Note the central pale staining macrophages (below) and the orderly peripheral rims of lymphocytes (above). (*H and E × 20*)

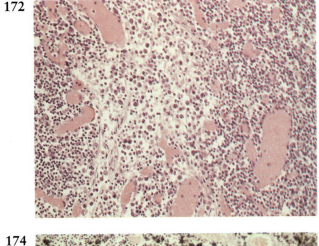

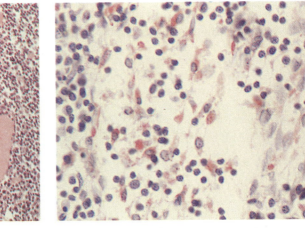

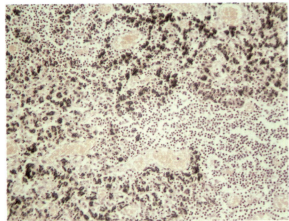

172 Proliferating macrophages in a sinusoid of a lymph node (centre). These cells often lie along the wall of the sinusoid, are called littoral cells and are phagocytic. (*H and E × 10*)

173 Phagocytosis. Lymph node from an animal injected with the red dye carmine. It has been phagocytosed by the sinusoidal cells. (*H and E × 40*)

174 Phagocytosis of black carbon pigment by macrophages in a lymph node. This is a common feature of lymph nodes draining the lung. (*H and E × 10*)

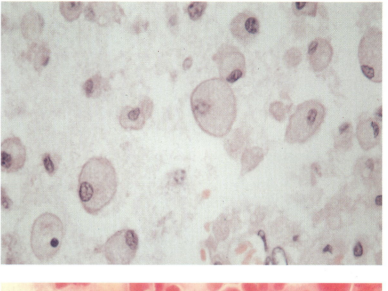

175 Large, bloated macrophages adjacent to an area of brain damage. These are microglial cells, often called Gitterzellen. (*H and E × 20*)

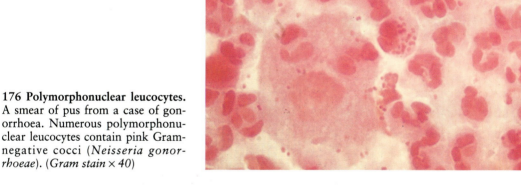

176 Polymorphonuclear leucocytes. A smear of pus from a case of gonorrhoea. Numerous polymorphonuclear leucocytes contain pink Gram-negative cocci (*Neisseria gonorrhoeae*). (*Gram stain × 40*)

Acute inflammation

Irrespective of the cause, inflammation occurs whenever cells die or are injured, provided that blood circulation continues in their vicinity. In simple creatures, like starfish larvae, with no vascular system, inflammation consists of an accumulation of phagocytes. Development of the vascular system, particularly in homoiotherms, has caused this basically simple process to become exceedingly complex.

For example, inflamed skin is hot, red, swollen and painful, and one is disinclined to move it. These are the cardinal features of inflammation, and most can be explained in terms of the microscopic findings.

The first event in tissue injury is transient arteriolar constriction, followed rapidly by conspicuous and prolonged vasodilatation, mainly of capillaries and venules. This is mediated by a variety of vasoactive substances that come from plasma, damaged cells and platelets. These dilated vessels may have such a sluggish flow that the blood clots within them (thrombosis). Vasoactive substances cause vasodilatation, and increase the permeability of the vessels. They affect the contractile elements in endothelial cells and in the pericytes that surround the capillaries and venules, opening the gaps between endothelial cells. Histamine is a vasodilator compound found in mast cells and in blood basophil leucocytes. It is released when an antigen reacts with immunoglobulin E in, for example, hypersensitivity reactions (q.v.). Serotonin (5-hydroxytryptamine) in blood platelets also causes increased vascular permeability. Derivatives of the complement components C3 and C5 (called C3a and C5a, or anaphylotoxins) are also potent mediators of vascular permeability. Protein derivatives such as bradykinin and kallikrein also play a part. Prostaglandins derived from polyunsaturated fatty acids are also important mediators (see Further reading).

In those vessels that have not thrombosed, leucocytes move to the peripheral plasmatic zone, stick to the endothelial surface, and migrate between the endothelial cells leaving the vessels and entering the inflamed connective tissues (**177**). Vasoactive substances aid in attracting leucocytes out of vessels and in promoting increased permeability. Chemotactic factors are responsible for the migration of neutrophil and eosinophil leucocytes and monocytes into sites of inflammation. Most important of these are C3a (anaphylotoxin) and the soluble complement complex C5, C6, C7.

Others include kallikrein and peptides derived from fibrin, collagen and bacteria. Prostaglandins play no part in chemotaxis.

Plasma and red cells also exude from the dilated vessels, and the resultant fluid and cells that appear in the connective tissues is called an inflammatory exudate. If the exudate is caused by bacterial action, the organisms may continue to proliferate. Many of the phagocytes and tissue cells may be killed by the bacterial toxins, and the resultant necrotic material is called pus (**178–189**). Death of cells in inflammation is also caused by hydrolases released from lysosomes in phagocytes. Pus bordered by an inflammatory reaction is called an abscess. It may be acute, as we have described here, or it may last much longer, when it is said to be a chronic abscess. An abscess in a hair follicle is called a boil. It bursts because the tension inside it stretches the overlying epidermis that becomes ischaemic and dies. When the boil bursts, pus is released and healing begins. The healing phase is called chronic inflammation and comes on about 48 hours after the start of an uncomplicated acute inflammatory response.

177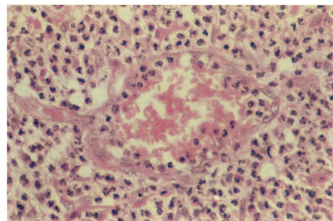

177 Acute inflammation. A capillary surrounded by polymorphonuclear leucocytes in an area of inflammation in the lung. Leucocytes are adherent to the vascular endothelium (margination), from here they will migrate into the surrounding tissue. (*H and E × 20*)

178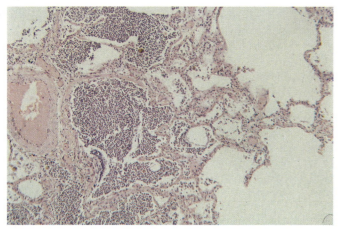

178 Purulent exudate in some alveoli of the lung (left) from a case of bronchopneumonia (q.v.). Alveoli to the right are dilated as a compensatory measure for the obstruction of alveoli on the left. (*H and E × 4*)

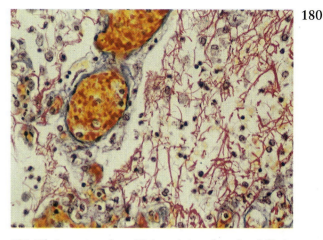

179 Alveolar exudate. Higher power view showing leucocytes in the alveoli together with strands of fibrin. Venules in the alveolar walls are dilated as part of the inflammatory response. (*H and E × 10*)

180 Fibrinous exudate. Pink staining threads of fibrin with leucocytes in alveoli. The vessels are dilated. (*McFarlane's modification of Mallory's trichrome method × 20*)

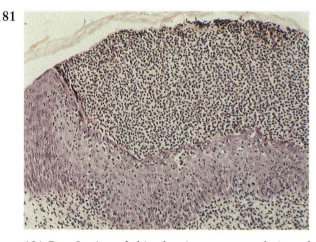

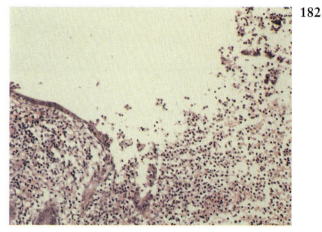

181 Pus. Section of skin showing an accumulation of pus (pustule) in the epidermis. This is often seen in impetigo which is a superficial infection caused by coccal bacteria. (*H and E × 10*)

182 Purulent exudate. The edge of an ulcer in the colon. Damaged colonic epithelium is seen on the left and purulent exudate in the base of the ulcer on the right. (*H and E × 4*)

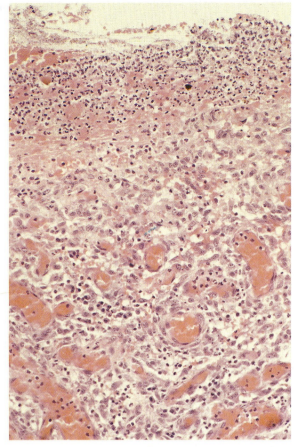

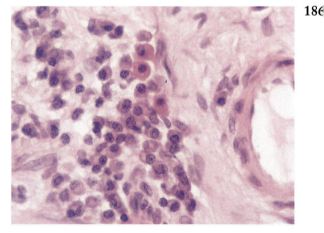

183 Fibrinopurulent exudate. The wall of an ulcer showing fibrinopurulent exudate on the surface (top) and newly formed vessels (granulation tissue) deeper down. (*H and E × 10*)

184 Acute inflammation. Section of heart muscle and visceral pericardium showing a pink layer of fibrin on the surface. Inflammatory cells and dilated vessels are present in the underlying connective tissue. (*H and E × 10*)

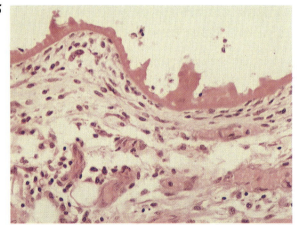

185 Acute inflammation. Higher power view of the visceral pericardium. Movement of the heart in the pericardial sac causes strands of fibrin to project into the lumen of the pericardial sac. This is called 'bread and butter' pericarditis, because a similar appearance occurs if two slices of buttered bread are pulled apart. (*H and E × 20*)

186 Plasma cells and mast cells adjacent to a capillary on the right. The few mast cells have a bright red cytoplasm. (*H and E × 40*)

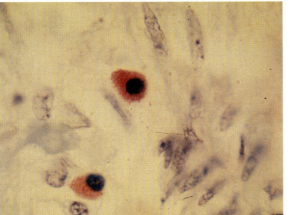

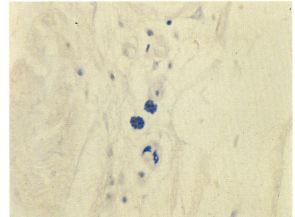

187 Mast cells with fibroblasts on the right. The mast cell granules have stained bright red with solachrome cyanin. (*Solachrome cyanin × 40*)

188 Mast cell granules also stain bright blue with toluidine blue, which stains the proteoglycan components, such as heparinoids in mast cells. (*Toluidine blue × 20*)

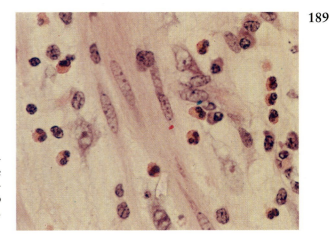

189 Eosinophil leucocytes scattered amongst lymphocytes in the wall of a vermiform appendix. They are often found in inflamed appendices and other gut derivatives, such as the gall bladder, and they have two nuclear lobes, unlike mast cells which have single nuclei. (*H and E × 40*)

Chronic inflammation

At about 48 hours after the inflammatory response has started fibroblasts appear; they are derived from fixed mesenchymal cells and they start to elaborate collagen. Young collagen is very like reticulin (2.7 nm periodicity) and it matures later to adult collagen (6.4 nm). If tension is intermittent, then elastic tissue forms as well as collagen (**190–192**). Vascularisation of the newly formed tissue is achieved by solid cords of endothelial cells that bud from adjacent capillaries, later becoming canalised and rejoining the parent vessel by forming a capillary loop.

A special situation exists in the central nervous system, where chronic inflammation is accompanied by a proliferation of the glial cells that are normally found there. Polymorphonuclear leucocytes are the principle phagocytes in the acute phase, but microglia appear in the chronic phase. These are usually inconspicuous cells with thin, flat nuclei. When these macrophages devour damaged brain tissue, they fill with droplets of lipid and are called Gitterzellen or compound granular corpuscles (**175**).

Chronic lesions in the central nervous system (CNS) do have collagen and fibroblasts in them because fibroblasts can get into the CNS from the connective sheaths of penetrating blood vessels. The principle cell, however, in chronic processes in the CNS is the astrocyte, which is a plump cell with a slightly eccentric nucleus. This is a glial cell and produces lots of glial fibres that are concerned with repair processes in the brain and spinal cord (**143, 193, 194**).

190

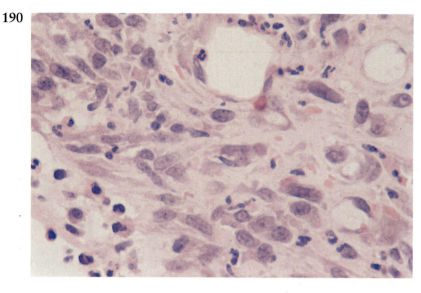

190 **Fibroblasts** adjacent to newly formed capillaries in a healing wound. (*H and E × 40*)

191

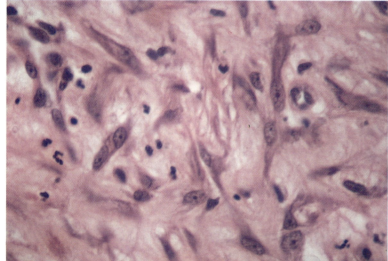

191 **Fibroblasts.** High power view showing the delicate nuclear chromatin and single nucleoli. The pink intracellular material is collagen. (*H and E × 40*)

192

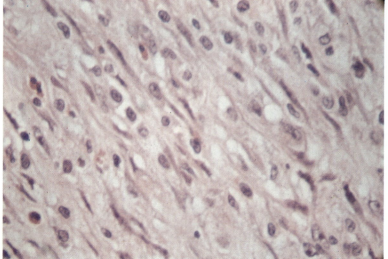

192 **Fibroblasts** aligned in rows in a healing wound. Lines of stress in a wound tend to produce this effect. (*H and E × 20*)

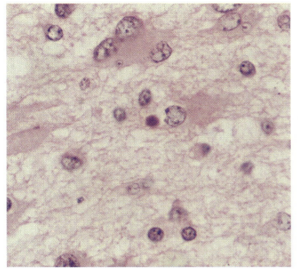

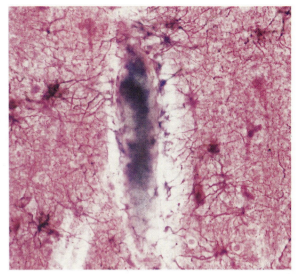

193 Plump astrocytes in the brain. These glial cells have abundant ragged cytoplasm and produce glial fibres which are part of the healing process in the central nervous system. (*H and E × 40*)

194 Astrocytes (star-shaped cells) around a central blood vessel. Their fine processes are shown by this method of staining. (*Cajal's gold sublimate × 20*)

Granulation tissue

A boil that bursts on the skin surface produces a break in the epidermal surface: any such break in an epithelial surface is called an ulcer. Viewed with a hand lens, the base of the ulcer consists of tiny red pin points; these are the newly formed capillary loops and have led to the name granulation tissue being applied to it.

Granulation tissue is composed of:

- Dilated and thrombosed vessels.
- Newly formed capillaries (**195–197**).
- Inflammatory exudate containing 'acute' inflammatory cells (e.g. polymorphonuclear leucocytes), and chronic inflammatory cells (such as fibroblasts, macrophages and lymphocytes), and later, as a result of the antigenic stimulus from the inflamed area, plasma cells. Quite often, binucleate plasma cells are found in chronic inflammatory processes, together with circular, amorphous pink Russell bodies that are probably related to antibody formation (**198–200**). **201–206** illustrate further examples of chronic inflammatory processes.

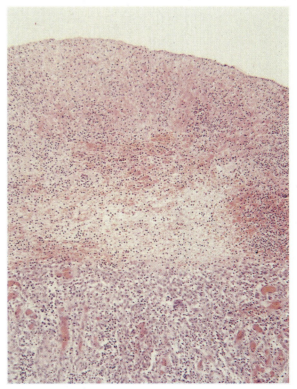

195 Granulation tissue. An ulcer showing fibrinopurulent exudate on the surface (top), and granulation tissue in the base composed of new capillaries and inflammatory cells. (*H and E × 10*)

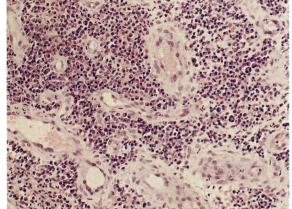

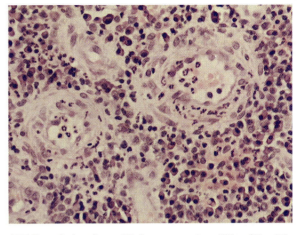

196 Granulation tissue showing newly formed capillaries with plump endothelial cells separated by sheets of plasma cells. (*H and E × 10*)

197 Granulation tissue. Higher power view. (*H and E × 20*)

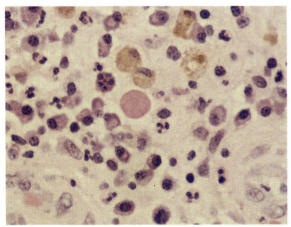

198 Granulation tissue. Plasma cells, fibroblasts and macrophages with pink cytoplasm in granulation tissue. (*H and E × 20*)

199 Granulation tissue. Plasma cells and Russell body (centre) in granulation tissue. Haemosiderin laden macrophages are also present. (*H and E × 40*)

200 Granulation tissue. Plasma cells, fibroblasts and macrophages in granulation tissue. Macrophages can sometimes be difficult to differentiate from mast cells. A special stain to show mast cell granules may be needed to make the distinction. (*H and E × 40*)

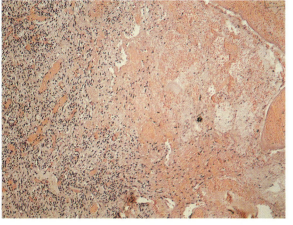

201 The edge of a pulmonary infarct. The necrotic tissue is on the right. The lung on the left shows a chronic inflammatory reaction to the dead tissue of the infarct. (*H and E × 4*)

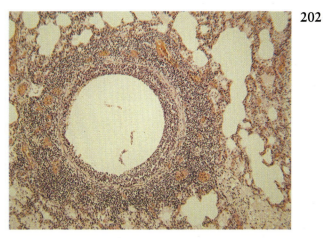

202 Bronchiole in a child's lung containing an acute inflammatory infiltrate. A dense chronic inflammatory reaction surrounds the bronchiole. (*H and E × 4*)

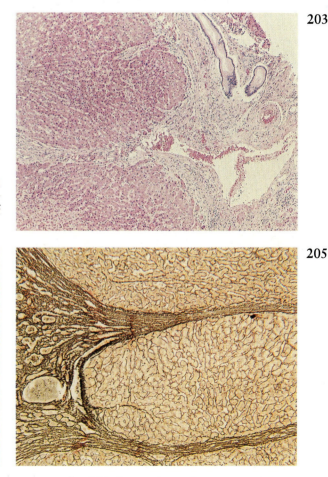

203 Liver damage. Section of liver showing a portal tract to the right, and two nodules of regenerative liver separated by collagen on the left. This is the end stage of liver damage causing nodular cirrhosis. (*H and E × 2*)

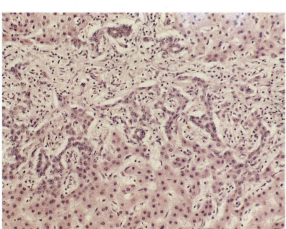

204 The edge of a cirrhotic nodule showing liver cells below, and a band of collagen bordered by regenerating cells which resemble bile ducts. (*H and E × 10*)

205 Strands of black reticulin and separate nodules of regenerate liver in cirrhosis. (*Gordon and Sweet × 4*)

206

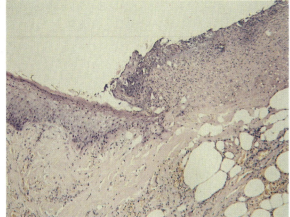

206 The edge of a chronic skin ulcer. The ulcer is to the right, with the epidermis to the left. The underlying dermis shows dense pink collagenous scar tissue which also embraces adipose tissue cells on the right. (*H and E × 4*)

Granuloma

Necrosis can be modified by the causative agent; the same applies to inflammation, so that it is sometimes possible, by looking at a section of an inflammatory process, to speculate upon what might be the cause of it.

Viral infections tend to produce a mononuclear response of macrophages and lymphoid cells rather than polymorphonuclear cells. Some bacteria produce a lot of pus and are said to be pyogenic (for example Staphylococcus and Streptococcus). Other bacteria, like *Salmonella typhi*, produce a chronic inflammatory response, and macrophages form the main component of the lesion (**207**).

Many organisms, particularly certain bacteria, fungi and metazoa, cause a nodular inflammatory response. The cells concerned are tightly packed and clearly circumscribed to form a lesion that is called a granuloma (**208–210**). It is not easy to define a granuloma, because it consists of various types of chronic inflammatory cells that appear in widely differing proportions in different diseases. The cells that are found in granulomas are:

- Macrophages.
- Lymphocytes.
- Plasma cells.
- Fibroblasts forming collagen.
- Giant cells.

As we have said, the proportions of these components vary greatly, and this variation may provide diagnostic histological criteria for the recognition of the cause of the granuloma.

Macrophages may constitute the sole feature of the granuloma in leprosy. Here the nodule, from the skin, consists solely of spindle-shaped cells packed with intracellular acid fast bacilli. Such closely packed macrophages come to resemble columnar epithelial cells, and are sometimes called epithelioid cells (q.v.). They are differentiated macrophages that have lost the ability to phagocytose, but can take up small particles by pinocytosis.

Lymphocytes are often present in granulomas, usually around the edge. Occasionally they form the bulk of the lesion, as in the nodules in the joints and lungs in rheumatoid disease and in mycoplasmal infections. In some of the autoallergic diseases, like Hashimoto's disease (q.v.), the thyroid is almost entirely replaced by lymphoid tissue, giving rise to the 'struma lymphomatosa' (**212, 213**).

Plasma cells are B lymphoid cells with a rich endoplasmic reticulum that have differentiated to the sole task of antibody production. Their cytological features have already been described. They occur predominantly in granulomas of the upper respiratory tract (middle ear, pharynx and tonsil), so much so that there is sometimes doubt whether these are neoplastic or granulomatous conditions. Plasma cells abound in chronic diseases such as syphilis, and binucleate plasma cells and Russell bodies are frequently present too.

Fibroblasts may form the bulk of fungal granulomas and granulomas that form around inert foreign particles, such as silicon dioxide in the lung (**211**). Seaweed extracts such as carrageenan are used experimentally to produce fibroblastic proliferations.

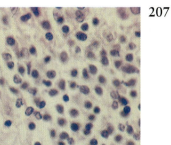

207 Granuloma. A cluster of pale staining macrophages with ill defined cytoplasm on the left. From a mesenteric lymph node in a case of typhoid fever. (*H and E × 20*)

208 Tuberculous granuloma with a pink caseous necrotic centre bordered by epithelioid macrophages in a lymph node. (*H and E × 4*)

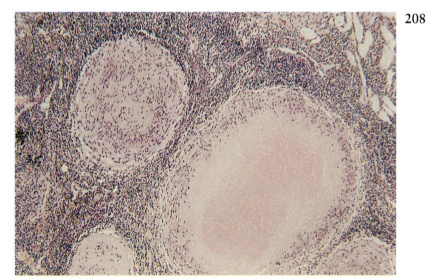

209 Schistosomal granuloma in the liver showing an egg in the centre surrounded by a pale zone of macrophages and an outermost zone of lymphocytes. (*H and E × 10*)

210

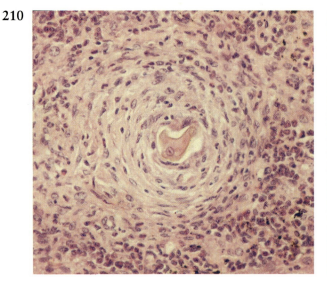

211

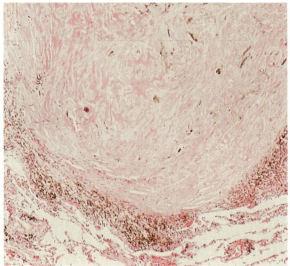

210 Schistosomal granuloma. A higher power view of **209** to show the cell detail. (*H and E × 20*)

211 A pink fibrous silicotic nodule with compressed lung tissue along its lower border. (*H and E × 2*)

212

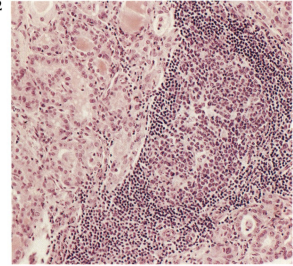

213

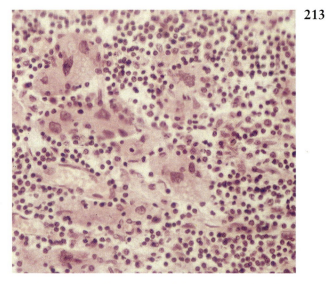

212 Thyroid showing a large central lymphoid focus, as is seen in Hashimoto's disease. (*H and E × 10*)

213 Lymphoid cells invade and distort thyroid cells in Hashimoto's disease. This is an autoallergic disorder where antibodies to thyroid tissue are found. The pale distorted thyroid cells are called Askanazy cells. (*H and E × 20*)

Giant cells

Giant cells appear in many kinds of granuloma. Originally, it was thought that specific sorts of giant cells were associated with particular diseases, but the more one looks at them the less likely this seems to be true (**214, 215**). Giant cells are formed either by the fusion of macrophages or by the division of macrophage nuclei without cytoplasmic cleavage: the former seems to be more likely. The simplest sort of giant cell forms around foreign body particles such as catgut, wood, etc. The foreign particle that elicits the reaction can often be seen in an ordinary H and E preparation viewed in visible light. Occasionally one has to resort to the use of polarised light. Here use is made of the ability of the crystalline foreign object to deflect the parallel rays of polarised light, so that the object shows brightly against a black ground. Any solid or liquid that has an orderly arrangement of molecules in it is able to deflect polarised light and is said to be anisotropic or birefringent (**216–219**).

Living and inert foreign agents cause giant cells to appear. Giant cells in tuberculosis are often large with nuclei scattered around the edge of the cells, and are called Langhan's giant cells. The peripheral nuclei in giant cells probably indicate a late stage in giant cell development. Cells with central nuclei are younger, recently formed cells. Fungi and viruses, notably herpes, respiratory syncytial virus and measles, occasionally cause giant cells to appear (**228**). Larger parasites such as metazoa have associated giant cells which are a reaction to the foreign material in the egg, larva or adult (**156**).

The classical granuloma is that seen in tuberculosis, where there is central necrosis and more peripheral epithelioid cells, giant cells and lymphocytes. Suitable staining methods (Ziehl Neelsen) demonstrate the organism as slightly curved red rods, sometimes finely beaded along their length and arranged in clumps.

Generally, the granuloma suggests to the histologist that some sort of hypersensitivity mechanism is operative. This is so in tuberculosis and in many other disorders, such as syphilis and the various sorts of arteritis (**229–232**).

One of the most mysterious granulomatous diseases is sarcoidosis (literally 'fleshy disease') where many parts of the reticulo-endothelial system are enlarged (lymph nodes, spleen, liver) and contain granulomas that are also present in other tissues, such as skin, bone, eyes, lungs, heart, etc. The cause of sarcoidosis is obscure, though some think that inhalation of pine pollen is a factor. Giant cells are a conspicuous feature of the granulomas of this disease and they contain a variety of structures. The granulomas are very like those of tuberculosis, but there is no central necrosis (caseation). Giant cells may contain globular bodies, asteroid bodies and Schaumann bodies (**233–237**), but none of these is specific for giant cells of sarcoidosis. In fact, the sarcoid granuloma is not specific for the recognition of sarcoidosis; such granulomas may be present in a variety of conditions (**220–227**):

- Around insect bites in the skin.
- In lymph nodes draining sites of carcinoma.
- In relation to blood shed into the tissues.
- In the lungs after inhalation of beryllium dust.
- In farmer's lung (James's lung) due to the inhalation of the fungus *Thermospora* from mouldy hay.

Granulomas are often found in the gut wall, notably in the ileum, colon and, to a lesser extent, stomach. They are associated with a chronic localised thickening of the gut, caused by diffuse chronic inflammation of the wall. This is called regional ileitis, regional colitis or Crohn's disease. The cause is obscure and granulomas appear late in the disease; again they may be due to repeated sensitisation of the injured gut wall by foreign material penetrating from the lumen of the gut.

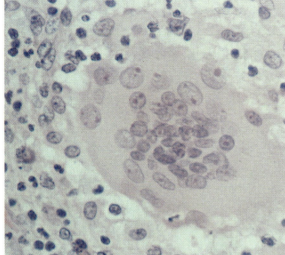

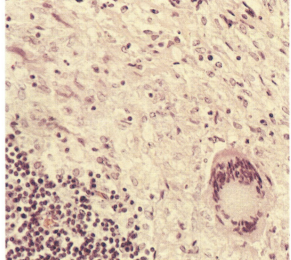

214 A typical giant cell with centrally arranged nuclei and peripheral macrophages and lymphocytes. This used to be called a foreign body giant cell, but it is not related to any specific stimulus. It is an example of a newly formed giant cell. (*H and E × 40*)

215 Langhan's giant cell in tuberculosis. The cell has peripherally arranged nuclei. The rest of the granuloma consists of epithelioid cells (right) and lymphocytes (bottom left). (*H and E × 20*)

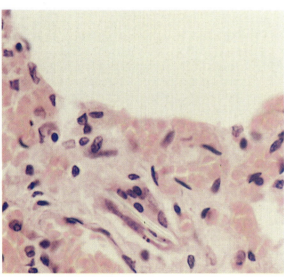

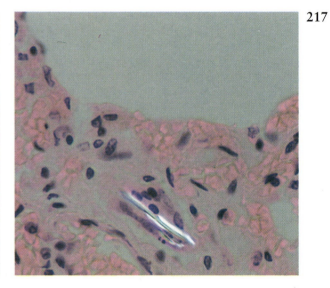

216 Foreign body. A sliver of foreign material in a lung capillary with a giant cell attached to it. From the lung of a drug addict who injected drugs intravenously. This is probably a piece of glass from a syringe. (*H and E × 40*)

217 Foreign body. The same section as **216**, viewed in polarised light. The foreign particle is birefringent within a giant cell. (*H and E polariser × 40*)

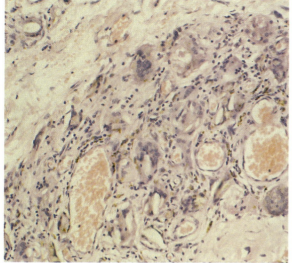

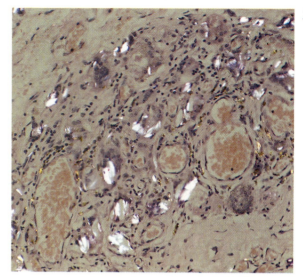

218 A foreign body giant cell reaction on the surface of an ovary. This is caused by glove powder shed into the peritoneal cavity at a previous operation. (*H and E × 10*)

219 Foreign body giant cell. The same section as **218**, viewed in polarised light. The talc particles are brilliantly birefringent. (*H and E polariser × 10*)

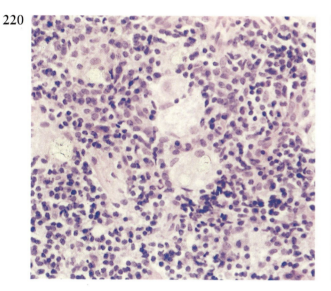

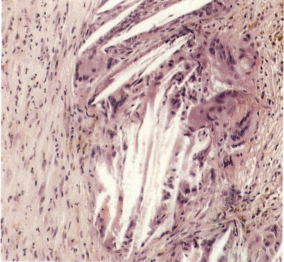

220 Giant cell. A lymph node containing giant cells which enclose particles of foreign material. This is material injected into the lymphatic circulation to make the lymph nodes visible radiographically, a technique called lymphangiography. (*H and E × 20*)

221 A giant cell response to cholesterol in an old haemorrhage. The cholesterol has been dissolved out of the section during paraffin embedding and is represented by the spindle-shaped spaces. (*H and E × 10*)

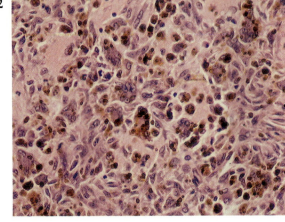

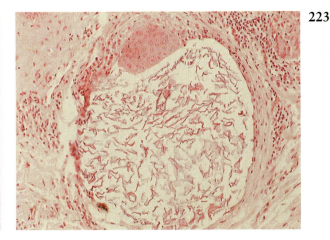

222 A giant cell response to brown haemosiderin pigment. This is seen in some benign skin tumours and in old haemorrhages. (*H and E × 20*)

223 A cyst in the skin containing pink flakes of keratin which have caused a foreign body giant cell to appear at the upper part of the cyst. (*H and E × 10*)

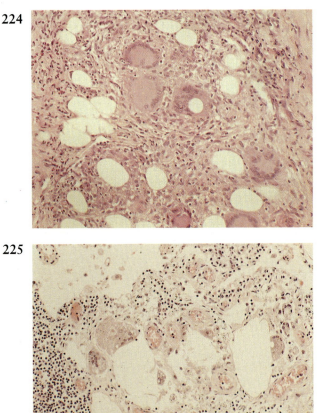

224 A giant cell response to necrotic fat. Some of the giant cells have globules that contained lipid. (*H and E × 10*)

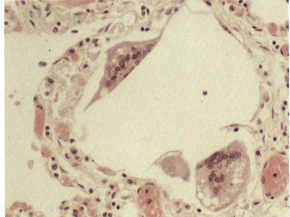

225 Lipid. Spaces that contained lipid in the lung. This has evoked a giant cell and chronic inflammatory reaction. Lipid, such as oily nasal drops, may produce this effect if inhaled into the lung. (*H and E × 10*)

226 Lipid. A space that contained lipid bordered by giant cells some of which contained lipid. The same case as **225**. (*H and E × 20*)

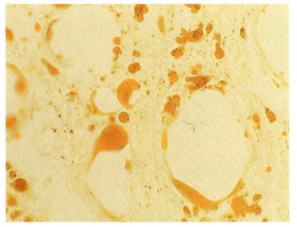

227 Fat. A frozen section (stained for fat) preserves the fat which is stained red. (*Oil red O × 20*)

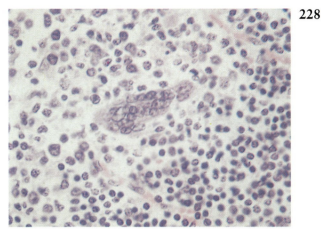

228 'Mulberry' giant cell from the spleen of a child infected with the measles virus. Giant cells are found in several viral infections. (*H and E × 20*)

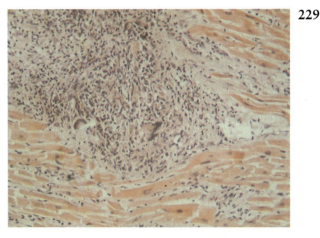

229 A granuloma containing giant cells in the heart. Sometimes this is due to sarcoidosis, but often the aetiology of giant celled myocarditis is unknown. (*H and E × 10*)

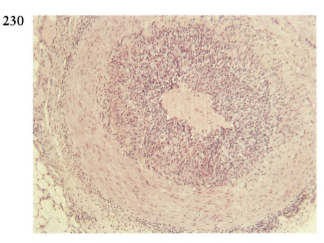

230 Giant celled arteritis showing a dense inflammatory response in the intima and related internal elastic lamina. Giant cells are sparse in this section. (*H and E × 4*)

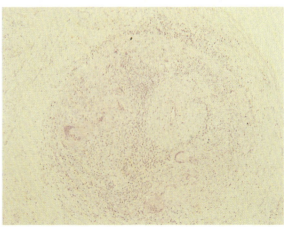

231 Giant celled arteritis showing giant cells in the inflammatory cells in the inner part of the artery. (*H and E × 4*)

232

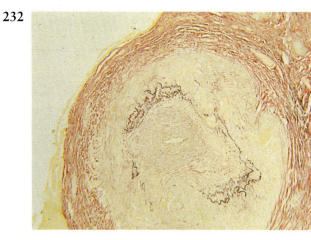

232 Giant celled arteritis. An artery showing loss of black elastic tissue of the internal elastic lamina. Giant celled arteritis destroys the arterial wall leading to thrombosis (q.v.). It is a connective tissue disorder but the precise cause is unknown. (*Weigert's resorcin fuchsin ponceau S × 4*)

233

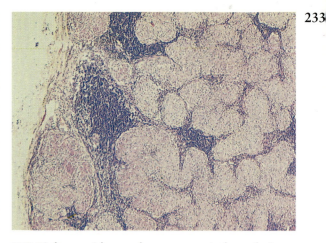

233 Pink sarcoid granulomas extensively replacing a lymph node. The nodules consist of epithelioid cells. There is no necrosis. (*H and E × 4*)

234

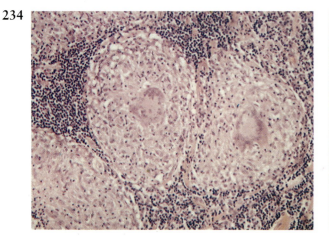

234 Sarcoid granulomas, higher power view. Giant cells are situated in nodules of epithelioid cells. There is no evidence of necrosis as is seen in the granuloma of tuberculosis. (*H and E × 10*)

235

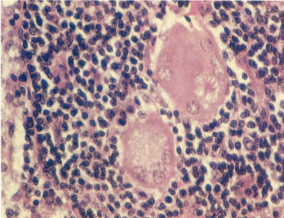

235 Two giant cells. The one below contains an asteroid body, the one above has globular bodies in the cytoplasm. (*H and E × 20*)

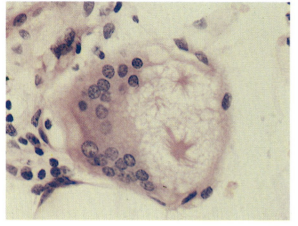

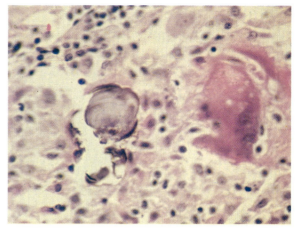

236 Giant cell containing red, star-shaped asteroid bodies and many globules. Asteroid and globular bodies are often seen in giant cells and are not specific to any disease process. (*H and E × 40*)

237 Schaumann body. A blue calcified body to the left (Schaumann body) which has come out of the giant cell to the right. This is also a non-specific inclusion in giant cells. (*H and E × 40*)

Repair and regeneration

Repair of a damaged tissue may follow the acute inflammatory process if the aggravating cause is eliminated or suppressed. We have already considered chronic inflammation and this is part of the repair process. Broadly repair consists of:

- Removal of necrotic debris (phagocytosis).
- Replacement of dead tissue either by collagen (repair by scarring) or by the appearance of new cells of the tissue to replace the damaged ones (regeneration).

Repair by scarring commonly occurs when highly specialised structures are destroyed. For example, a deep cut in the scalp heals by scarring, and this leaves a bald patch because the specialised hair follicles fail to regenerate in the scar (**238**). The less specialised epidermis is, however, capable of regeneration and grows over the surface of the scar, thus producing healing of the wound. Mitoses are often very frequent in such regenerating epidermis and it is important not to confuse this active normal tissue with a neoplasm (q.v.).

Liver readily regenerates after pieces have been excised or destroyed in some way. Again, abundant mitoses in the liver cells may give a false impression of neoplasia (**239**).

Some structures, like axons and skeletal muscle cells, are quite capable of regeneration, provided the neurilemmal and sarcolemmal tubules persist in the damaged tissue. If an axon is crushed but the neuron is intact then a new axon grows into the neurilemmal tube distal to the crushing. It follows that axonal regeneration does not occur in the central nervous system where there are no such neurilemmal structures. Crushed skeletal muscle behaves in the same way: new myoblasts and myofilaments appear from swollen sarcolemmal nuclei, and these fill the sarcolemmal tube. If the sarcolemma is transected, then a knot of newly formed myoblasts, with nowhere to go, forms yet another kind of giant cell; a muscle giant cell (**240**).

Factors concerned in regeneration are poorly understood. Regeneration of cells, such as those of the liver and skin, is accompanied by a burst of mitotic activity. When regeneration is complete, the cells of the tissue revert to the normal state of cell division. This regulation of growth is achieved by several factors. One is contact inhibition, that is, direct contact by one cell with another, which slows down cell division. This may be the result of the formation of intercellular junctions, allowing recognition molecules to pass from one cell to the other. In some neoplasms (q.v.) which continue to grow, such junctions are not formed. Inhibitors of cell multiplication are called chalones. These are balanced by stimulants of cell division called trephones or antichalones.

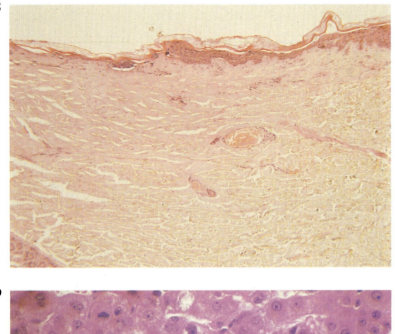

238 Scar. Thin epidermis overlying a dense pink collagenous scar, from a healed skin ulcer. (*H and E × 4*)

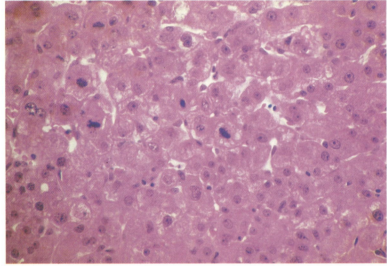

239 Liver regeneration. Section of liver from an area adjacent to resected liver. The black mitoses indicate liver regeneration. (*H and E × 20*)

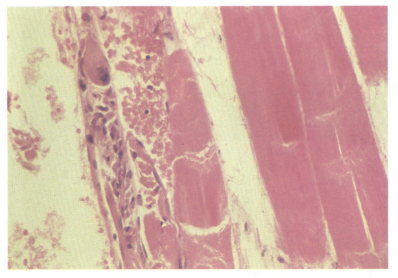

240 Muscle regeneration. Dead necrotic skeletal muscle on the right. On the left are proliferating sarcolemmal nuclei with occasional newly formed myoblasts. An example of muscle regeneration after injury. (*H and E × 20*)

7 Patterns of disease

Infection

Infections may remain confined to a particular organ in which they arise, or they may spread widely to produce septicaemia and death. For example, lung infections provide a diversity of reactions due to the differing properties of the agents that cause them. Bacterial infections may be pyogenic or not, as we have seen. Many bacteria that gain entry to the lung when the epithelial barriers are destroyed by cold, age, smoke or poisons, cause purulent infiltrations in the lung (**241, 242**). These occur in the bronchioles and in the adjacent alveoli, usually in the dependent lower lobes of the lungs. The condition is called bronchopneumonia and is often preceded by bronchitis (bronchial and bronchiolar inflammation) (**243**).

Bronchopneumonia is, then, a patchy process scattered throughout the lower lobes. Adjacent alveoli may be collapsed because the respiratory bronchiole is blocked by pus from the bronchopneumonic area. Other alveoli may be compensatorily dilated (emphysema) (**244**). Appearances in bronchopneumonia vary according to the nature of the organism and its virulence. Staphylococci may cause haemorrhagic pneumonia where much blood is present in alveoli; this is an effect of the alpha toxin (**123–126**). Occasionally, if the virulence of the organism is high, the bronchopneumonic areas may coalesce so that the whole lobe is involved (confluent bronchopneumonia), and intense necrosis in such a lobe may lead to abscess formation. If the patient recovers, the exudate in the alveoli may organise. This is a progressive process characterised by fibroblasts entering the alveolar exudate, and ultimately filling the alveoli with fibrous tissue (**245, 246**).

Lobar pneumonia is a different disease. It is usually caused by a pneumococcus and is peculiar because the whole lobe or lobule of the lung is uniformly involved, right from the start of the process. The disease progresses in stages over a period of about eight days, after which the patient may recover completely and dramatically. Early on, the changes in the alveoli are those of acute inflammation: the alveolar exudate contains fibrin, erythrocytes and abundant pneumococci. Later, the character of the exudate changes, becoming more purulent and the pneumococci disappear (**247**). Later still, macrophages appear to clear away the intra-alveolar debris, and the lung returns to normal. An exudate of fibrin always appears on the pleural surface in lobar pneumonia, because the whole lobe is uniformly involved. This uniform involvement is one of the mysteries of lobar pneumonia and may be due to a hypersensitivity mechanism (q.v.). Mechanisms responsible for the hypoxia, toxaemia crisis, and death in this disease are poorly understood. Toxins secreted by bacteria, pneumolysin or teichoic acid from bacterial breakdown or other substances may also be factors in the pathogenesis of lobar pneumonia.

A wide variety of bacteria may cause acute purulent bronchitis and bronchopneumonia; these are infections that either kill the patient or are resolved in a matter of days. More chronic, long-standing disorders of the lung are caused by organisms such as fungi and mycobacteria; the best known of these is tuberculosis. In children, this leads to caseation in the lung (Ghon focus) and in the draining lymph node: the two lesions are called the primary complex. A similar lesion occurs in the ileum and its related lymph nodes, caused by *Mycobacterium tuberculosis* swallowed in infected milk or swallowed in infected sputum from a lung lesion (**250–252**). In the adult, the lung lesion is better confined by a fibrous capsule and its spread to the local lymph node does not occur. Some think that this is due to the protective hypersensitivity conferred by the primary infection of childhood.

If either primary (childhood) or secondary (adult) lesions rupture into a bronchus, they give rise to tuberculous bronchopneumonia (**248, 249**). If they rupture into a branch of the pulmonary artery, then tuberculous material is spread over the body causing small tuberculous granulomas in many organs (kidney, liver, spleen, adrenals, meninges). This is called miliary tuberculosis and was a uniformly fatal disorder before the advent of tuberculostatic drugs (**253, 254**). Miliary tuberculosis is an example of septicaemic spread of *M. tuberculosis* from a local lesion in the lung or from local lesions elsewhere in the body.

241

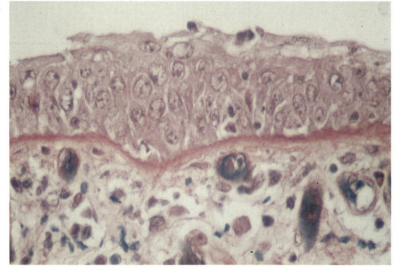

241 Squamous metaplasia, caused by the inhalation of irritants such as tobacco smoke, impairs the ciliary clearance mechanisms in the bronchial tree and predisposes to bronchitis and bronchopneumonia. The surface epithelium has been transformed into a prickle cell layer resembling epidermis. (*Mallory's phosphotungstic acid haematoxylin × 20*)

242

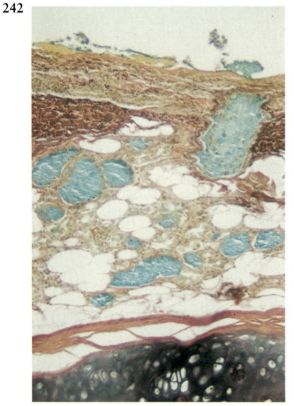

242 Mucous glands in a section of bronchial wall. The glands stain green, they are enlarged and produce abundant green mucus which is spreading on to the surface. Increased mucous gland activity is a feature of chronic bronchitis. (*Alcian blue × 4*)

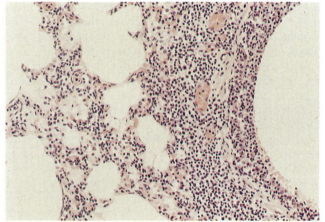

243

243 Acute purulent bronchitis. The lumen of the bronchiole (right) is lined by purulent exudate. Inflammatory cells are also present in the adjacent lung tissue. (*H and E × 10*)

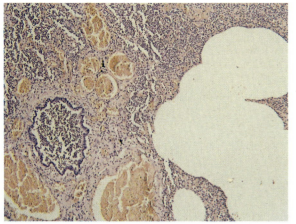

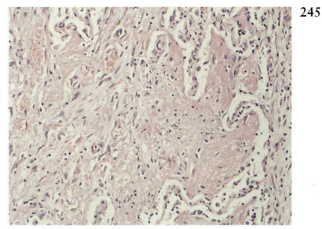

244 Bronchopneumonia. Pus is present in a bronchiole (left) and in the surrounding alveoli. The large space on the right is compensatory emphysema. This is overdilatation of alveoli adjacent to others that are consolidated. (*H and E × 4*)

245 Bronchopneumonia. Lung showing fibrinopurulent exudate of bronchopneumonia which is organising by fibroblasts. (*H and E × 10*)

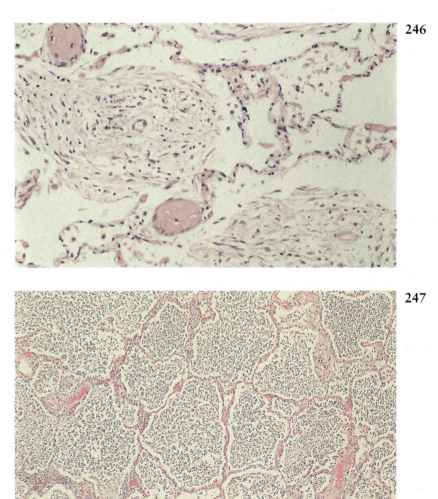

246 Bronchopneumonia. Alveoli containing delicate strands of pink collagen and fibroblasts from organising bronchopneumonia. (*H and E × 10*)

247 Lobar pneumonia. Alveoli uniformly filled with polymorphonuclear leucocytes from a case of lobar pneumonia. Capillaries in the alveolar wall are dilated. There is no damage to the alveolar walls themselves. (*H and E × 4*)

248

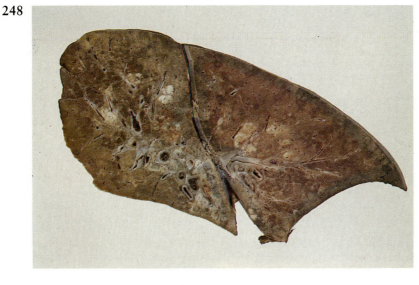

248 Tuberculous bronchopneumonia. A slice of lung showing white caseous areas of tuberculous bronchopneumonia. This occurs when caseous material from a primary focus in the lung erupts into a bronchus and is inhaled into the air passages.

249

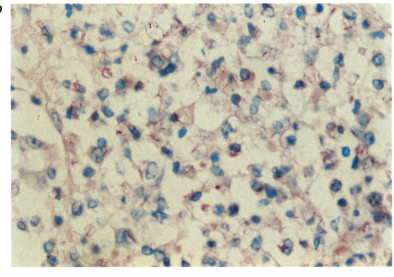

249 Tuberculous bronchopneumonia. Large numbers of red acid–alcohol fast tubercle bacilli in the exudate from the case of tuberculous bronchopneumonia in **248**. (*Ziehl Neelsen × 40*)

250

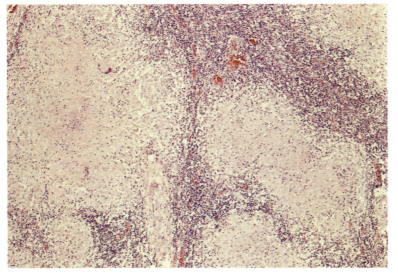

250 Tuberculous follicles in a lymph node draining a tuberculous lesion in the lung. Note the pink caseous necrosis and giant cells. (*H and E × 2*)

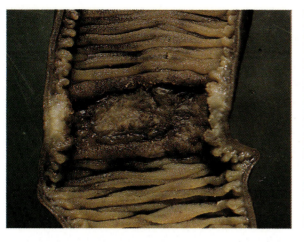

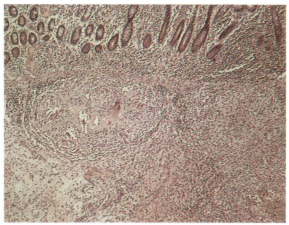

251 Typical transverse tuberculous ulcer in the ileum. The lesion is transverse because the organism spreads around the gut wall in the lymphatics. Note the white caseous foci in the gut wall on either side of the ulcer.

252 Section of the ileum shown in **251** showing the epithelium above and caseous foci in the subjacent submucosa. (*H and E × 2*)

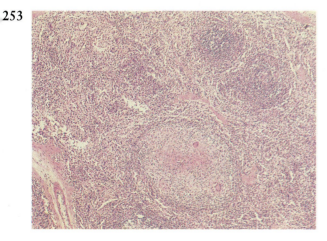

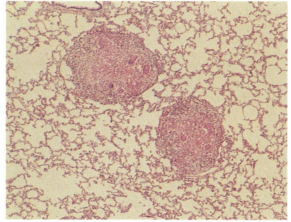

253 Miliary tubercle in a spleen, with adjacent Malpighian bodies. (*H and E × 4*)

254 Miliary tubercles in a child's lung. (*H and E × 4*)

Trauma

There is a steady increase in the incidence of traumatic injury on the roads in the UK, and also as a result of violence in modern society. A study of traumatic lesions is important, particularly to the forensic pathologist, for it often enables the cause and time of the injury to be determined.

The presence of an inflammatory reaction at the edges of a wound obviously indicates that it was sustained before death. The demonstration of haemosiderin in a bruise indicates that the bruise is at least 48 hours old, for haemosiderin takes that time to form (255–258).

Heat coagulation of tissue at the edge of a wound can be spotted microscopically. If there is also a blackening of the wound, this suggests that a cartridge has been discharged at close range, as in a suicidal shooting, and enables the nature of the missile to be suspected (261, 262).

By the application of general knowledge of the processes of inflammation, it is possible to determine the age of a wound fairly accurately. This is an important issue in forensic pathology. For example, the recognition of the battered child syndrome, where a child is repeatedly beaten and may ultimately die, may rest upon the determination of wounds of various ages on and within the body. Skin bruising and haemorrhage into various organs may be found in these children. Haemorrhage that occurs over and in the brain and in the eye may cause disability in later life if the child survives (263).

Bones are frequently involved in traumatic injury. The process of healing in bone is similar to healing elsewhere in the body, but is complicated by the appearance of specialised tissues and by the use of redundant terminology. Bone is either compactly arranged, as in the cortex of long bones, or loosely arranged as a meshwork, as in the marrow space (compact and cancellous bone respectively). In the adult, both types are lamellar bone, consisting of layers of calcified collagen separating rows of osteocytes in lacunae (264). Because of its ordered arrangement, lamellar bone is birefringent. When new bone forms, as a result of fracture or other disorder, it is not laid down in an orderly way initially. It consists of irregularly arranged osteocytes enclosed in randomly distributed fibres, like the arrangement of strands in a ball of string. Such tissue is called woven bone and is not birefringent (265, 266).

Initially, a healing fracture shows a swelling on the bone, the primary callus. This is composed of fibroblasts, woven bone and variable amounts of cartilage depending on the degree of movement at the fracture site: the greater the mobility of the fracture, the greater the amount of cartilage (267, 268). Secondary callus is the complete restoration of the bone shape and continuity, by the transformation of woven to lamellar bone; this occurs by the combined action of phagocytic osteoclasts and osteoblasts that produce bone.

Extensive bony injury, for example, multiple fracture of ribs during attempted resuscitation, leads to the liberation of bone marrow into the venous circulation, and particles may be seen in sections of pulmonary artery (bone marrow embolism (q.v.) (271–273)).

In the elderly, or where extensive fractures occur in the young, fat may be liberated into the venous circulation, causing blockage of lung capillaries. Alternatively, it may pass by arteriovenous anastomosis to capillaries in the brain, kidney and heart, causing severe dysfunction there. Similar fat embolism may follow trauma to subcutaneous fat and other fatty tissues independent of that found in the adult bones (274–279).

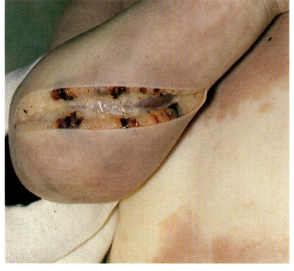

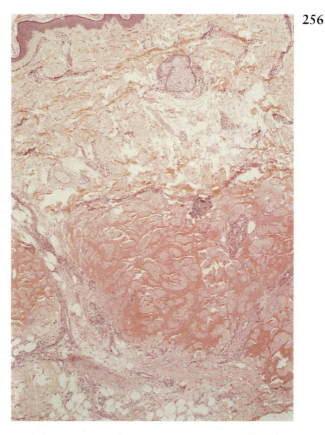

255 Trauma. Fresh, recent bruises on the upper arm of a battered child. They are readily seen in the incised subcutaneous fat, but are not easily shown on the skin surface. The purple colour indicates that the bruises are recent.

256 Section of a recent skin bruise showing blood deep in the subcutaneous tissue. Such bruises do not appear readily on the skin surface. (*H and E × 2*)

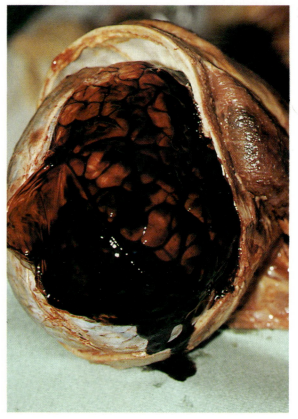

257 Subdural haemorrhage. View of the brain from above with the dura reflected, showing a subdural haemorrhage. This is caused by tearing of the small vessels running from the brain to the dura, following blows to the head.

258

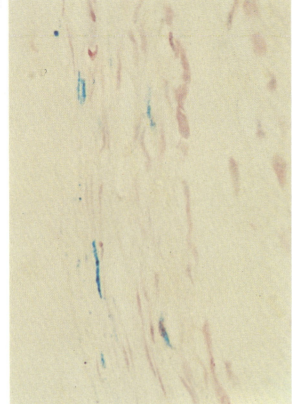

259

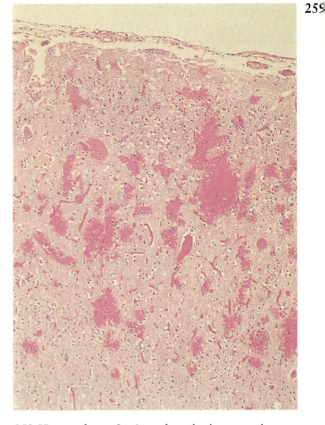

258 Subdural haemorrhage. Section of dura mater overlying a subdural haemorrhage. The dura (left) contains blue iron containing macrophages indicating that the haemorrhage had occurred several hours before death. (*Perls' stain × 40*)

259 Haemorrhage. Section of cerebral cortex, the surface is above. Multiple haemorrhages in the cortex, caused by vibration of the brain following head injury. (*H and E × 4*)

260

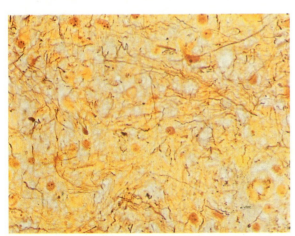

261

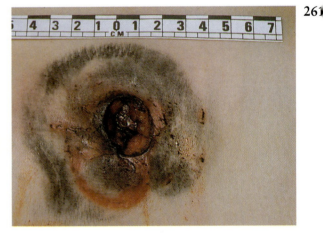

260 Concussion. Temporary loss of consciousness (concussion) may follow head injury. In such cases the brain may look normal to the naked eye. A section and a special stain will reveal broken axons which have retracted into small balls, shown black in this section. (*Silver stain × 40*)

261 Gunshot wound produced by the discharge of a 12 bore gun at close range. Note the abraded red impression of the undischarged barrel below, and the blackening of the wound produced by point blank discharge.

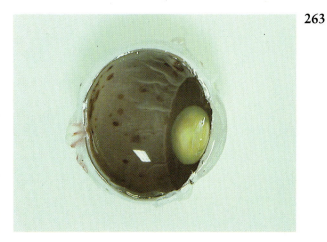

262 The edge of a gunshot wound in the skin. The epidermis is compressed, the dermis shows a uniform pink effect of heat coagulation, and powder is present at the edge of the wound (left). (*H and E × 10*)

263 Multiple haemorrhages in a transected eye from a child who died of non-accidental injury.

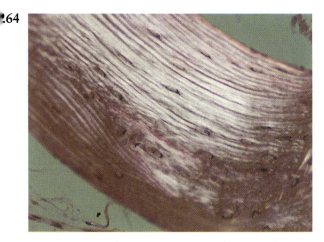

264 Lamellar bone showing the parallel array of collagen fibres with flat, regularly arranged osteocytes. (*H and E × 20*)

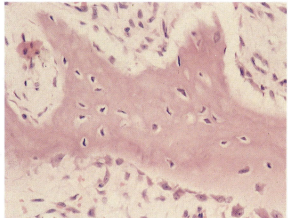

265 A piece of woven bone in a fracture. The osteocytes of woven bone are plump and irregularly arranged, unlike lamellar bone. (*H and E × 10*)

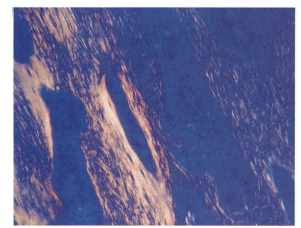

266 Bone. Birefringent lamellar bone on the left. The woven bone on the right is seen faintly, because of its lack of birefringence. (*H and E polariser × 4*)

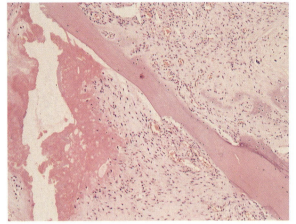

267 Section through a fracture site. The fracture is seen on the left as a gap containing fibrin. A strip of lamellar bone crosses the field obliquely and new, woven bone has formed on the right. (*H and E × 4*)

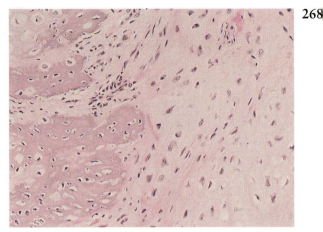

268 Fracture. If there is movement at the fracture site during healing, as in a rib, cartilage (right) as well as woven bone (left) appears in the callus. (*H and E × 10*)

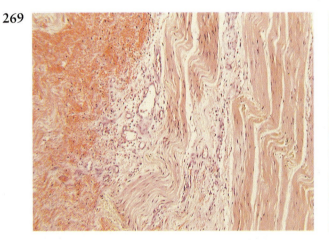

269 Fracture. Stretched and torn skeletal muscle (right) in the region of a bone fracture. There is haemorrhage into the muscle (left). (*H and E × 4*)

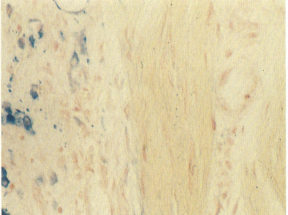

270 Fracture. The haemorrhage in the muscle (left) contains blue staining haemosiderin indicating that it is some hours old. (*Perls' stain × 20*)

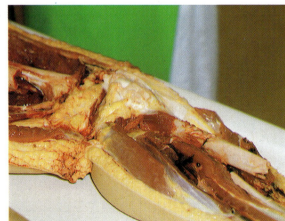

271 Fractures of the femur (left) and tibia showing haemorrhage into the muscle. Such fractures may cause the release of fat and bone marrow from the medullary cavity of the bone into the venous system. Such fragments finish up in the lung as bone marrow embolism.

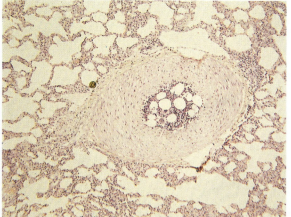

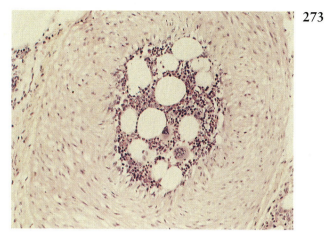

272 Bone marrow embolism. Section of lung showing fat and marrow in a pulmonary vessel. This is bone marrow embolism and it often follows rib fractures produced by attempts at resuscitation. (*H and E × 4*)

273 Bone marrow embolism. Higher power view of the embolus in 272 showing fat and bone marrow which contains two megakaryocytes. (*H and E × 10*)

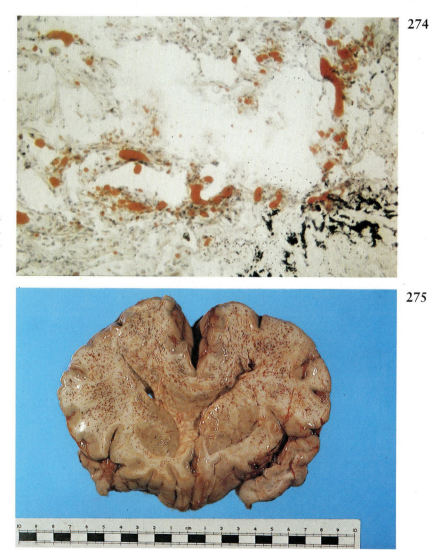

274 Fat embolism. Frozen section of lung showing red staining fat in pulmonary vessels. There is carbon pigment in the lung, bottom right. (*Oil red O × 4*)

275 Fat embolism. A slice of brain showing multiple small haemorrhages from a case of fat embolism. Particles of fat escape through the lungs into the systemic circulation.

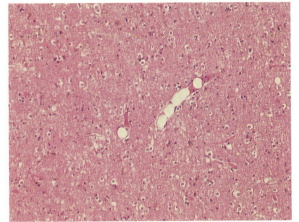

276 Globules of fat in cerebral capillaries. (*H and E × 10*)

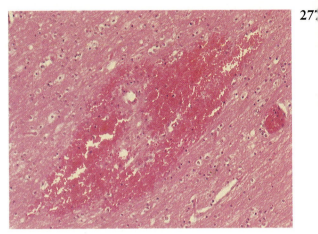

277 **Small haemorrhage** around capillaries obstructed by fat which cause the capillaries to leak blood. (*H and E × 10*)

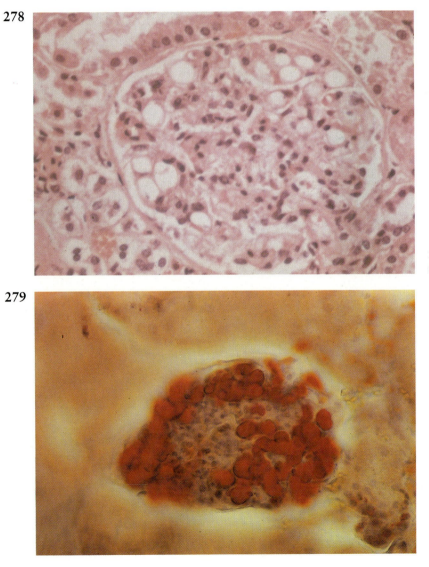

278 **Globules of fat in a glomerulus from fat embolism.** (*H and E × 20*)

279 **Fat embolism.** A thick frozen section of kidney showing glomerular capillaries distended by fat globules. (*Oil red O × 20*)

Ischaemia

Thrombosis

Ischaemia means literally 'to hold back blood'. It is a state where insufficient oxygen gets to the tissues. The causes are vascular obstructions of various kinds:

- Vascular disease leading to narrowing.
- Thrombosis.
- Mechanical obstruction such as
    Pressure
    Ligation
    Embolism, i.e. blockage by particles of material circulating in blood.

We shall deal, in this chapter, with thrombosis, which is really a sort of mechanical obstruction and worthy of consideration separately.

Blood clots when it becomes stagnant, but this is not thrombosis. A thrombus is an orderly structure made up of layers of platelets, fibrin and red blood cells. The fact that it is layered suggests that it forms as blood flows over the surface, that is, it forms in a living vessel (**280–286**).

Two factors are needed before thrombosis occurs:

- Injury to the vascular endothelium.
- Slowing of the blood flow in the vessel.

An increase in blood viscosity, due to either fluid loss or cellular increase, particularly of platelets, will further encourage the tendency for thrombi to form.

Several things may happen to thrombi:

- They may be removed by phagocytes or be dissolved by fibrinolysis.
- They may propagate so as to block the vessel and its branches.
- They may organise by the ingrowth of granulation tissue, and the vessel may ultimately be filled with a fibrous scar (**287, 288**).
- They may canalise and the vessel lumen is restored to some extent by cracks forming in the thrombus being lined by endothelium, or by the complete penetration of the blockage by newly formed capillaries (**289**).
- Infection of a thrombus may cause it to fragment and liberate particles of infected material into the circulation (pyaemia).
- A sterile thrombus in a vein may also break loose and impact in a pulmonary artery (pulmonary embolism).

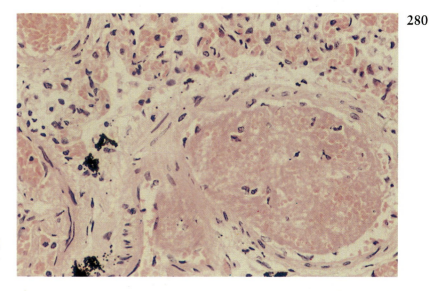

280

280 Recent thrombus, composed mainly of platelets and fibrin, in a pulmonary artery branch. (*H and E × 20*)

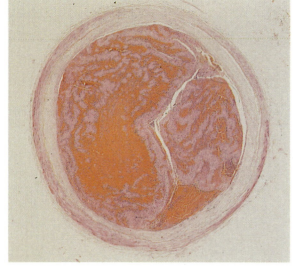

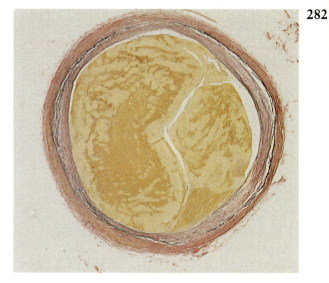

281 Thrombus. Low power view of an artery distended by recent thrombus. Note the deep red blood trapped between pink layers of platelets and fibrin. (*H and E × 2*)

282 Thrombus. A stain for elastic tissue and collagen shows the layers of the thrombus. This is a recent thrombus and there is no pink collagen in it. (*Weigert's resorcin fuchsin ponceau S × 2*)

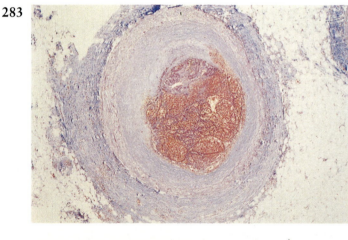

283 Thrombus. A trichrome stain shows platelets blue, red cells and fibrin red in this recent thrombus. (*McFarlane's modification of Mallory's trichrome stain × 2*)

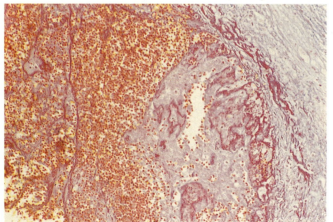

284 Thrombus. Higher power view of a thrombus showing deep red erythrocytes, blue platelets and red fibrin. (*McFarlane's modification of Mallory's trichrome stain × 10*)

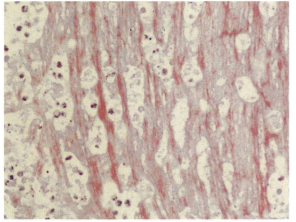

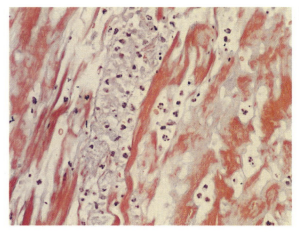

285 Thrombus consisting mainly of platelets and red fibrin in layers. Such thrombi are seen more often in arteries than in veins. (*McFarlane's modification of Mallory's trichrome stain × 20*)

286 Thrombus composed mainly of fibrin with a few platelets containing leucocyte nuclei. (*McFarlane's modification of Mallory's trichrome stain × 20*)

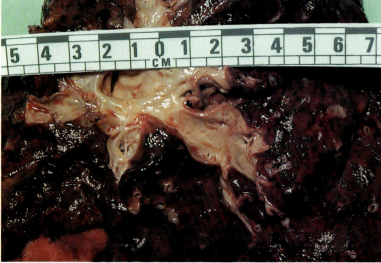

287 Thrombi. Pulmonary artery of lung opened to show strands of collagen in the lumen (middle of the picture). These fibrous strands are organised thrombi.

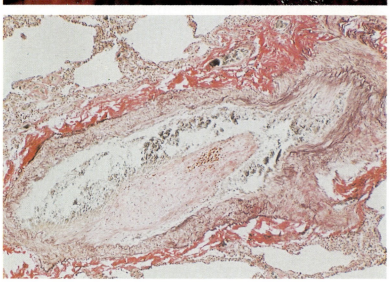

288 Thrombus. Low power view of a pulmonary artery branch containing a pink staining organised thrombus. (*Weigert's resorcin fuchsin ponceau S × 4*)

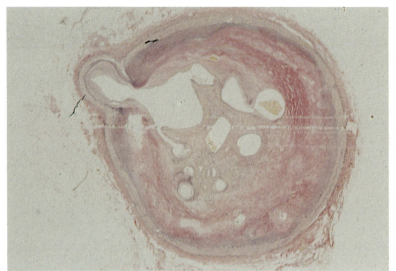

289 An organised thrombus in an artery which has consequently recanalised with the formation of new blood channels through it. (*Weigert's resorcin fuchsin ponceau S × 2*)

Embolism and infarction

Blockage of an artery or a vein may be due to emboli which may be thrombi, air, fat, neoplasms, parasites, foreign bodies and so on. The effects of air embolism (**290–293**) are similar to those of fat embolism.

The result of vascular blockage is determined by:
- The territory that the vessel supplies.
- The extent of the collateral circulation.
- The state of the collateral vessels – whether they are diseased or not.
- The rate of flow of blood through these vessels.
- The oxygen-carrying power of the blood that is depleted when the haemoglobin level is reduced (anaemia).
- The nature and activity of the tissue supplied by the vessel.

When part of an organ becomes ischaemic it dies; the dead tissue shows all the histololgical features of necrosis. At the edge of the dead tissue is a zone of acute inflammation, from which exudate pours into the necrotic area, causing it to become stuffed with exudate and inflammatory cells (infarction). An infarct, then, is an area of ischaemic necrosis. Some infarcts are pale yellow, others deep red. The colour depends on the vascularity of the structure; if there are many leaking vessels at the edge of an infarct, as in the lung, it is red. If the blood supply is radial, as in the kidney, then the infarct is pale. Infarcts caused by venous block are consequently often red wherever they occur (**294–298**).

An infarct, like any other inflammatory area, may organise and turn into a sunken scar.

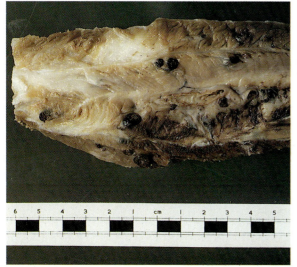

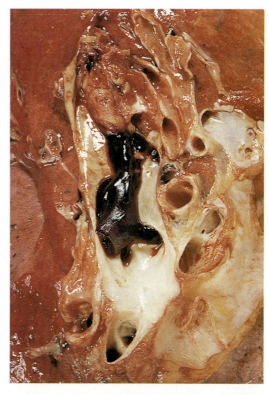

290 Dark coloured thrombi in a slice of calf veins. They may provide a source of pulmonary embolism.

291 Venous thrombus which has embolised into the main pulmonary artery. It is dark purple in colour because of its high content of red cells: a feature of venous thrombi.

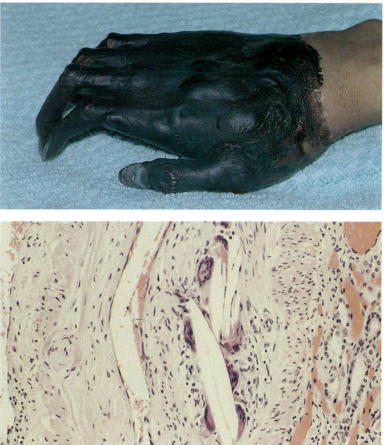

292 Gangrene of a hand. Most of the hand consists of dead black tissue. This is caused by an embolus into the brachial artery.

292

293 An embolus composed of cholesterol clefts and giant cells in a renal artery branch. This embolus usually comes from severe aortic atheroma. (*H and E × 20*)

293

294

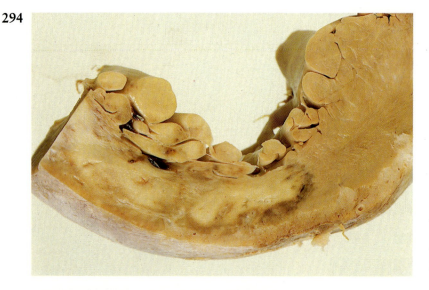

294 Infarction. Slice of left ventricle showing a pale yellow area of infarction bordered by a dark rim of inflammation which is a response to the necrotic tissue.

295

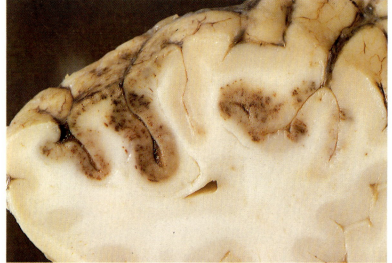

295 Infarction. A slice of cerebral cortex showing infarction of the grey matter (above). The cellular grey matter is more vulnerable than the white matter to ischaemia. Reduction of cerebral blood flow may result in this selective ribbon-like infarction.

296

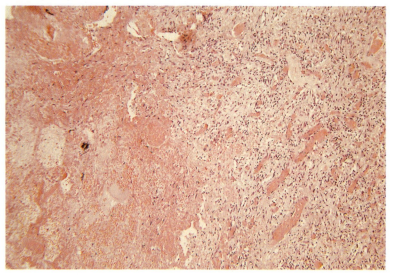

296 Area of infarcted lung tissue. Haemorrhage from adjacent vessels produces a red infarct in the lung. (*H and E × 4*)

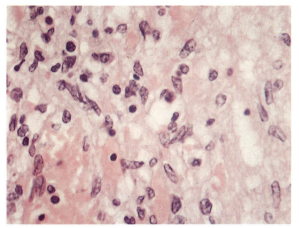

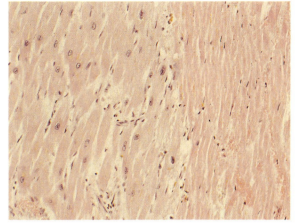

297 Edge of a splenic infarct (right). The less specialised cells of connective tissue have survived the ischaemia. (*H and E × 20*)

298 Edge of a myocardial infarct showing dead acellular myocardial fibres (right) and surviving nucleate fibres (left). (*H and E × 10*)

Hypoxia

If ischaemia is gradual, as may occur with progressive arteriosclerosis in organs such as the heart, kidney and brain, then the tissue affected shrinks gradually and is slowly replaced by fibrous tissue (**299, 300**).

Ischaemia causes local hypoxia. General hypoxia occurs when the oxygen supply to cells is reduced. This is seen in anaemia, when fatty change may occur in a variety of organs, such as the heart and liver. If the hypoxia persists then the cells die (**301, 302**).

Anaemia is due to blood loss, red cell lysis or inadequate red cell formation. The histological features in anaemia are often not conspicuous. If lysis is the cause, then abundant haemosiderin collects in the liver and spleen. This is also seen in some examples of inadequate red cell formation when iron is not being used up (**303**).

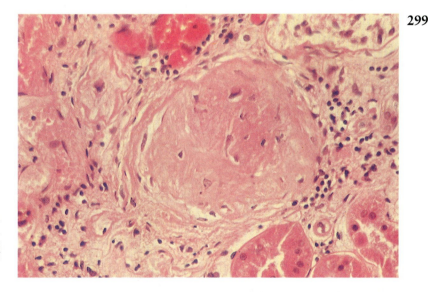

299 Hypoxia. A glomerulus which has been subjected to ischaemia from progressive arterial narrowing has become converted into a ball of fibrous tissue. (*H and E × 20*)

300

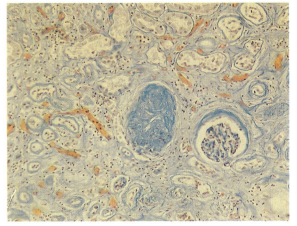

300 Hypoxia. Hyaline blue staining collagen replacing an ischaemic glomerulus. The early changes of ischaemia are seen in the adjacent glomerulus which shows collagenous thickening of the parietal layer of Bowman's capsule. (*McFarlane's modification of Mallory's trichrome stain × 10*)

301 Anaemia. Inner aspect of the right ventricle below the tricuspid valve showing mottled yellow strips of fatty change. This is called 'thrush's breast mottling' and occurs in severe anaemia.

301

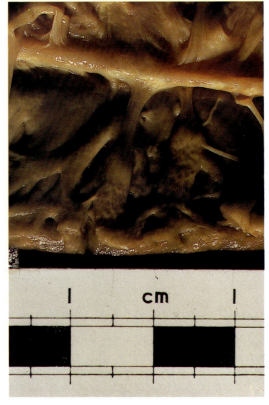

302

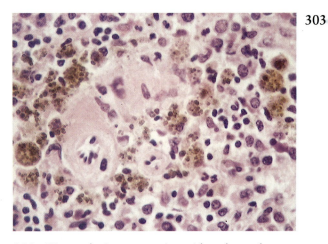

302 Anaemia. Subcapsular fatty change in the liver in an anaemic patient. (*McFarlane's modification of Mallory's trichrome stain × 10*)

303

303 Haemolytic anaemia. Abundant brown haemosiderin laden macrophages around a splenic arteriole from a case of haemolytic anaemia. (*H and E × 20*)

Ageing and arteriosclerosis

Degeneration is an unfortunate term implying progressive collapse of the fabric of the body with age. It is true that a variety of events come on with age. The bones become fragile and lose their trabeculae (osteoporosis). The collagen of the dermis fragments and takes up stains for elastic tissue ('senile' elastosis): this change occurs on the facial skin and may not necessarily be the result of age, but due to prolonged solar exposure (304–306). Lipochrome pigment collects in the liver, heart and neurons of the aged. Cerebral vessels become encrusted with iron and calcium, and the media of thyroid, uterine, ovarian and other vessels tend to calcify. Other age changes affecting the supporting tissues are seen in the bones. Elderly women may develop thin bones, a condition called osteoporosis. The supporting trabeculae within long bones, vertebrae and elsewhere are reduced in numbers and become thin. Such bones tend to fracture easily. This is a feature of age, but may also be related to oestrogen deficiency (307–309).

Probably the most important event that progresses with age is the gradual narrowing of many blood vessels by intimal thickening. This is one form of arteriosclerosis, which is a generic, nonspecific term for several kinds of arterial thickening. Arteriosclerosis comprises:

- *Intimal* fibro-elastic and muscular thickening seen in small arteries (310–312).
- *Atherosclerosis* which starts as an intimal accumulation of lipids, collagen and elastic fibrils and smooth muscle cells. Later the media is affected. This is a disease of large arteries (313).
- *Mönckeberg's sclerosis* which is a relatively unimportant medial calcification of the long arteries of the limbs. It has little effect on the vascular lumen (314).
- Various sorts of *vasculitis*, acute and chronic, seen in hypersensitivity disorders (315–317).

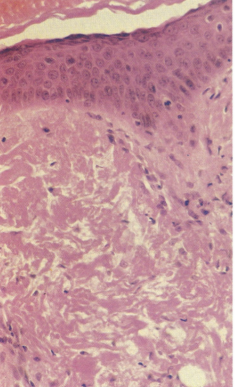

304 Skin showing thickening and fragmentation of dermal collagen. This feature of aged skin is aggravated by exposure to the sun and is called solar elastosis. (*H and E × 10*)

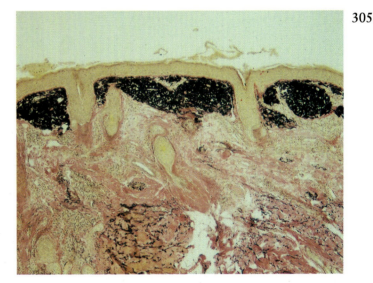

305

305 Degenerate collagen in the dermis stains black with stains for elastic tissue. It is called solar elastosis but the fibres are collagenous. (*Weigert's resorcin fuchsin ponceau S × 4*)

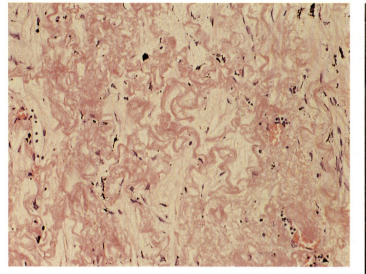

306 Collagen fibres in old scars in the lung show similar changes to those of solar elastosis. Such collagenous changes have many causes. (*H and E × 10*)

307 Vertebral slice from an elderly woman showing the sparse, thin trabeculae in the vertebral bodies.

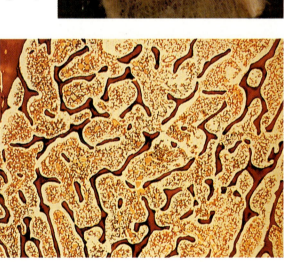

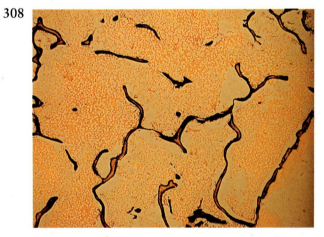

308 Section of osteoporotic bone showing thin, sparse trabeculae. (*Von Kossa × 4*)

309 Section of a normal vertebra for comparison with 308. (*Von Kossa × 4*)

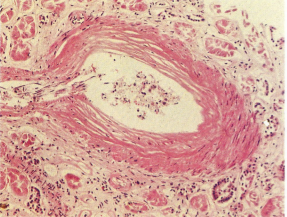

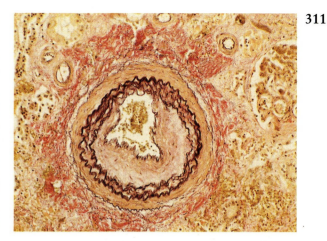

310 Intimal thickening of a renal arcuate artery and its branch (left). (*H and E × 4*)

311 A renal arcuate artery showing proliferation of elastic tissue (black) and pink collagen on its luminal side. (*Weigert's resorcin fuchsin ponceau S × 10*)

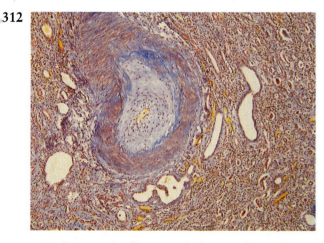

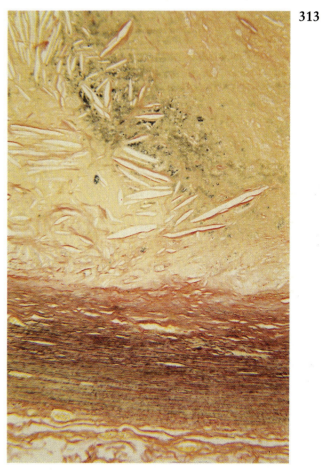

312 Blue intimal collagenous thickening of a renal arcuate artery. The elastic tissue also stains blue. (*McFarlane's modification of Mallory's trichrome stain × 4*)

313 An atheromatous plaque. The intima (above) is greatly thickened and contains cholesterol clefts and black flecks of calcium. The inner media (below) is partly replaced by pink collagen. (*Weigert's resorcin fuchsin ponceau S × 4*)

314

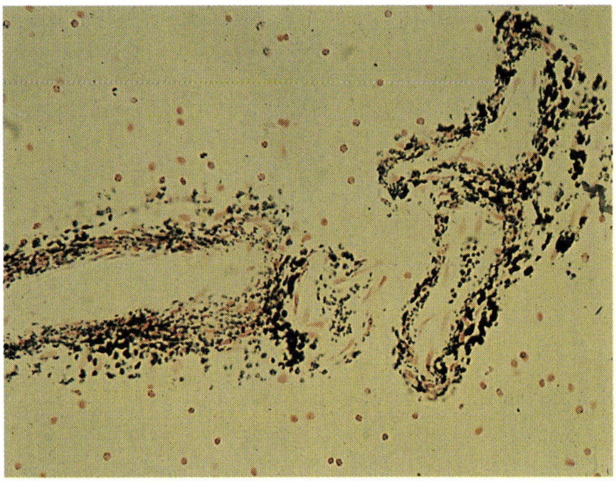

314 Medial calcification of cerebral blood vessels. The calcium is black (*Von Kossa* × *20*)

315

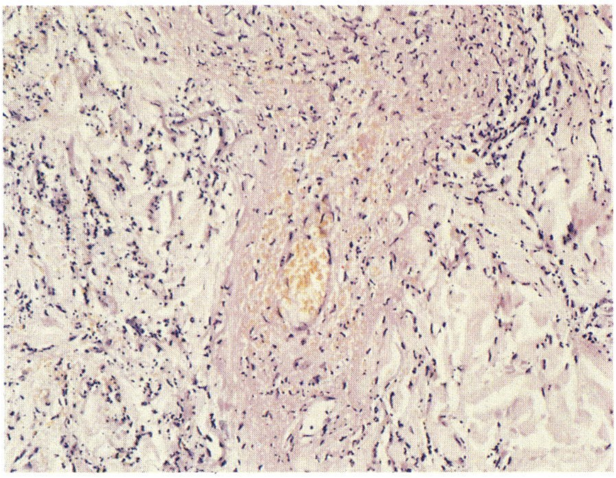

315 Acute vasculitis in the skin. The pink staining vessel is necrotic and infiltrated by inflammatory cells. Similar cells surround the necrotic vessel. Cutaneous vasculitis is an immune disorder. (*H and E* × *10*)

316

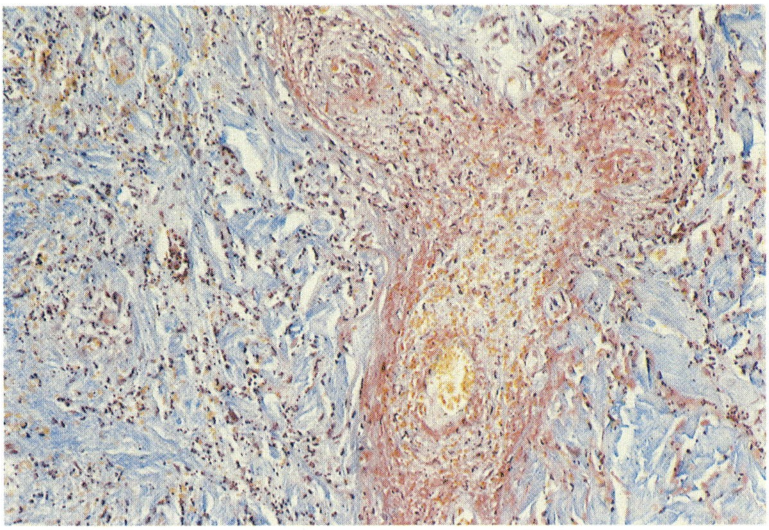

316 Acute vasculitis. Fibrin, leucocytes and red cells are present in the necrotic vessel wall. (*McFarlane's modification of Mallory's trichrome stain* × *10*)

317

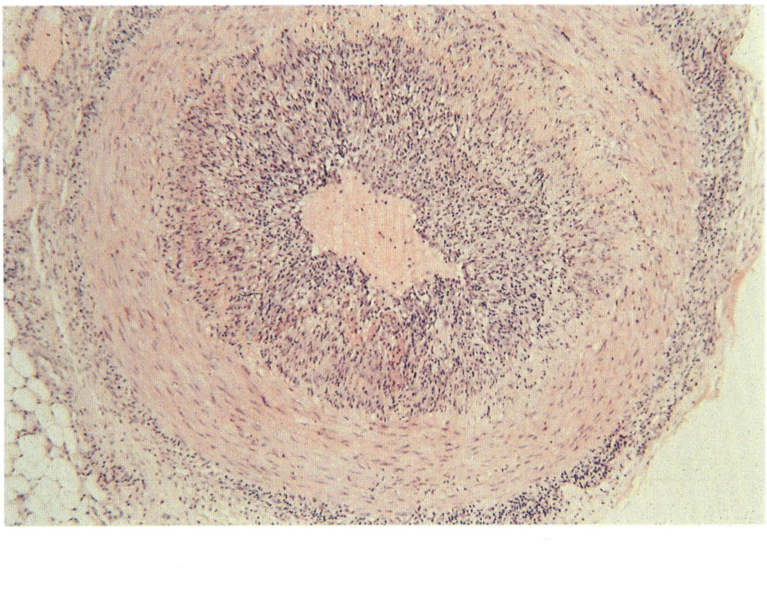

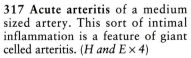

317 Acute arteritis of a medium sized artery. This sort of intimal inflammation is a feature of giant celled arteritis. (*H and E* × *4*)

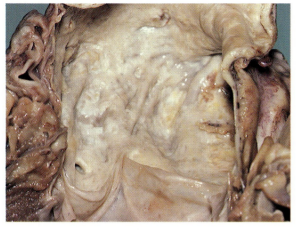

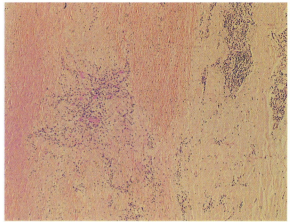

318 Syphilitic aortitis. Internal view of the ascending aorta from a case of syphilis. The aortic wall is grey and scarred.

319 Syphilitic aortitis. Granulation tissue in the aortic media (left). The adventitia (right) shows cuffing of blood vessels by lymphocytes and plasma cells. These are the appearances of syphilitic aortitis. (*H and E × 4*)

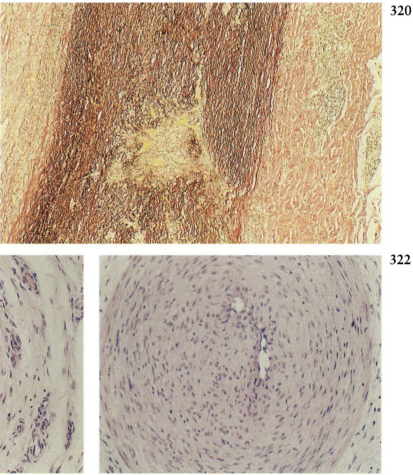

320 Syphilitic aortitis. Destruction of elastic tissue (centre) in syphilitic aortitis. This leads to aneurysm formation. (*Weigert's resorcin fuchsin ponceau S × 4*)

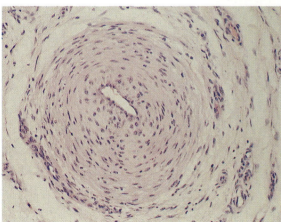

321 Syphilitic aortitis. Proliferation of endothelial and smooth muscle cells, obliterating the lumen of an artery in the adventitia. (*H and E × 10*)

322 Endarteritis obliterans, high power view. This process leads to vessel wall ischaemia, scarring and aneurysm formation. (*H and E × 20*)

Atherosclerosis

Atherosclerosis, or atheroma, is a common disease of large and medium sized blood vessels. It affects the aorta and its principal branches and, in particular, the coronary arteries, where it provides the commonest cause of death in the Western world. It is a progressive process of intimal thickening, which ultimately may occlude the involved artery or lead to thrombosis of the vessel, which is then occluded. It starts in childhood, and is seen in the coronary arteries and in the carotid sinuses. The earliest process is intimal thickening, due to smooth muscle and elastic tissue proliferation (323). Later, lipid brought in by macrophages collects in the lesion, and lesions called fatty streaks and spots are now visible in the vessels with the naked eye (324–329).

The lesions enlarge as the years go by, and collagen forms within them produced by smooth muscle cells (330, 331). Clefts of cholesterol are present, foci of calcification occur and the lumen of the artery is progressively narrowed (332–334). When the endothelial covering of the intimal lesion is breached, thrombosis occurs (335). When this occurs in the coronary arteries, the usual result is a cardiac infarct.

As well as intimal changes, there are also alterations in the media. These are produced because the intimal thickening leads to medial hypoxia and medial cell death. The result is partial replacement of the media by collagen, and the strength of the media is reduced. In the aorta, this leads to outward bulging of the vessel, causing an abnormal dilatation called an aneurysm. Such aneurysms in the abdominal aorta commonly rupture, leading to death.

Syphilis also causes aortic aneurysms, again by medial damage. In this case, the damage is due to progressive blockage of the vasa vasorum which supply the outer media (318–320). The intimal proliferation of these vessels is a common feature of many chronic infective processes, like syphilis and tuberculosis. Most of the proliferating cells are of endothelial or smooth muscle origin (321, 322).

The cause of atherosclerosis is unknown. It is mainly a human disease, though it has been found in other primates, aged birds and pigs. Several predisposing factors, including high blood pressure, smoking, high levels of blood lipids (such as lipoproteins and cholesterol), and diabetes mellitus are known (338). Other factors may be responsible, but their modes of action are not clearly defined.

The disease can be produced in a variety of experimental animals by feeding fats, raising blood pressure and other techniques. Considerable argument exists about the similarity of the animal to the human lesions. Basically, however, atherosclerosis is a smooth muscle cell proliferation in the arterial wall, as a response to injury of various sorts (339–346).

323

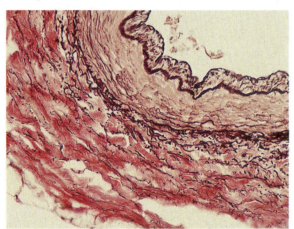

323 Atherosclerosis. The earliest detectable lesion of atherosclerosis in a child's coronary artery, showing elastic intimal thickening containing smooth muscle cells. (*Weigert's resorcin fuchsin ponceau S × 20*)

324

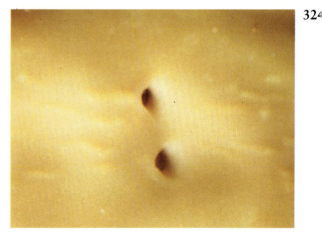

324 Fatty streaks in the thoracic aorta adjacent to the origins of intercostal arteries.

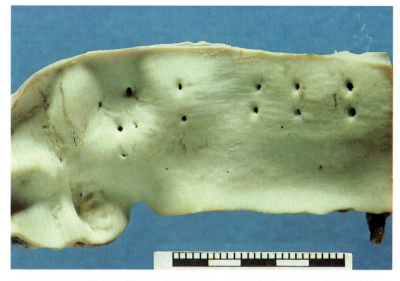

325

325 Fatty streaks in the thoracic aorta. They are barely visible.

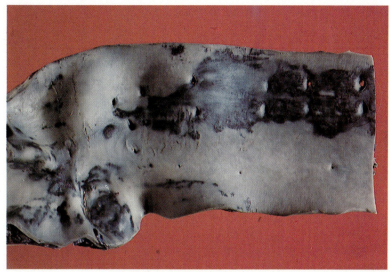

326

326 Fatty streaks. When the aorta is stained to show the fat content of the fatty streaks they are readily seen. (*Sudan black stain*)

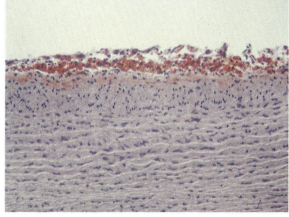

327

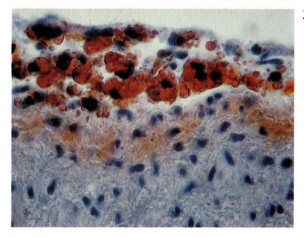

328

327 Section of a fatty streak showing the red staining lipid largely confined to the intimal surface. (*Oil red O × 4*)

328 Fatty streak, high power view. Most of the red staining lipid is in the macrophages, some is also extra-cellular. (*Oil red O × 20*)

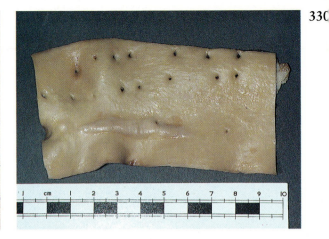

329 Fatty streak showing the spindle-shaped nuclei of smooth muscle cells in the lesion. (*H and E × 4*)

330 Linear fibrous plaque in the thoracic aorta. This is a later stage of development of the atherosclerotic lesion.

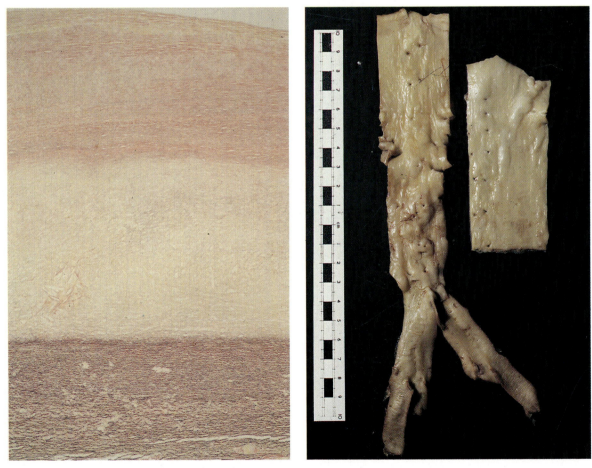

331 Fibrous plaque in a coronary artery. The lesion consists mainly of pink collagen (top) and lipid (middle). (*Weigert's resorcin fuchsin ponceau S × 2*)

332 Atherosclerosis. Thoracic aorta (right), abdominal aorta (left) showing nodular raised lesions of atherosclerosis. These are fibrous plaques that have accumulated lipid. The term atheroma is often confined to these lesions.

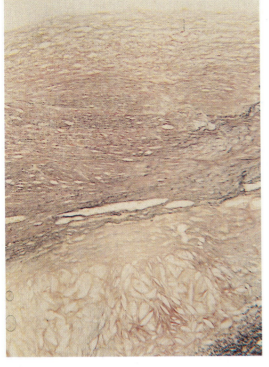

333 Section of an atheroma showing the fibrous cap over the top of the lesion and the accumulated lipid in the deeper parts (below). (*Weigert's resorcin fuchsin ponceau S × 4*)

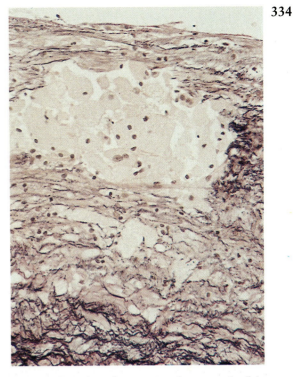

334 Lipid in the atheroma is often contained in foamy macrophages (top). (*Weigert's resorcin fuchsin ponceau S × 4*)

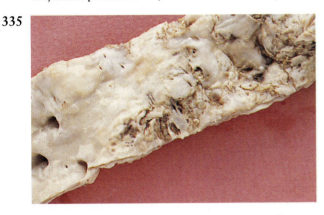

335 Abdominal aorta showing the end stage lesions. The surfaces of the lesion have ulcerated and thrombi have formed on them.

336 Iron is often found in aortic atherosclerotic lesions. This piece of aorta shows blue staining iron in the lesions. It is derived from ruptured small blood vessels that develop in the plaques.

337 Blue ferric iron (left and right) in an atherosclerotic plaque. Cholesterol spaces are towards the centre. (*Perls' stain × 4*)

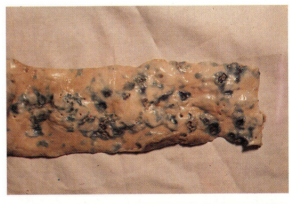

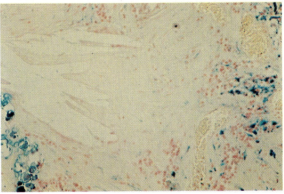

338

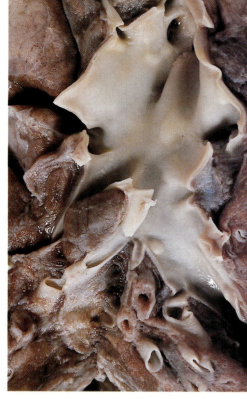

338 Plump yellow atheromatous plaques in the pulmonary artery of a child with a ventricular septal defect, which leads to a rise of pulmonary artery pressure and indicates the role of increased pressure in the production of atherosclerosis.

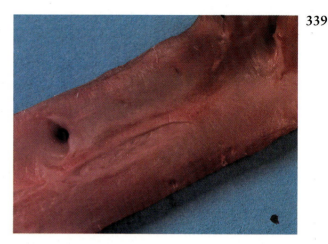

339

339 Naturally occuring atherosclerotic plaque in the aorta of a domestic turkey. It is a raised, linear lesion with red staining lipid at the edges. (*Oil red O*)

340

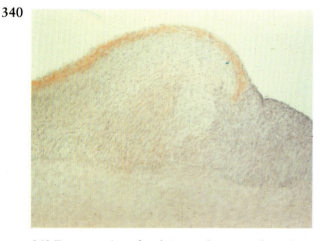

341

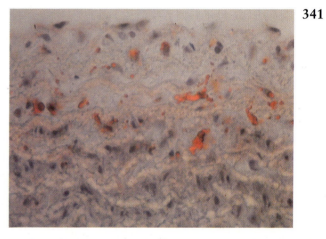

340 Frozen section of a plaque in the aorta of a turkey. Red staining surface lipid, overlying the lesion composed of smooth muscle. (*Oil red O × 4*)

341 Atherosclerosis. Frozen section of naturally occuring atherosclerosis of a domestic pig. Note the resemblance to the human fatty streak (**327**). (*Oil red O × 10*)

342 Experimentally induced atherosclerosis in the rabbit. The red lipid containing lesions are distal to the intercostal orifices. The lesions were produced by feeding cholesterol to the animal.

342

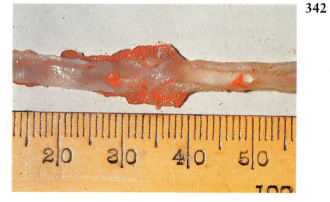

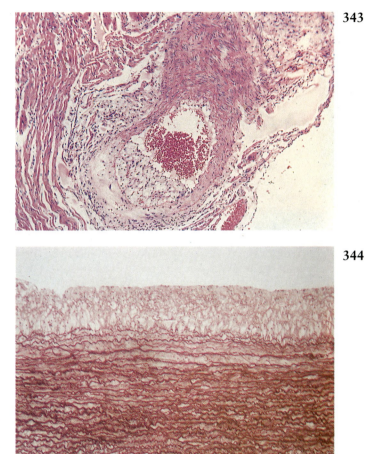

343

343 Experimental atherosclerosis. Rabbit coronary artery showing intimal macrophages (below). Such lipid laden cells are a feature of cholesterol induced atherosclerosis in the rabbit. (*H and E × 10*)

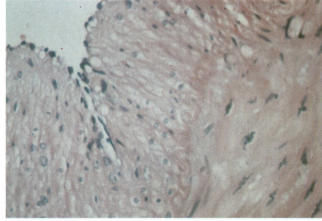

344

344 Experimental atherosclerosis in the rabbit aorta. The intima (top) is replaced by a layer of macrophages. (*Weigert's resorcin fuchsin poneau S × 4*)

345

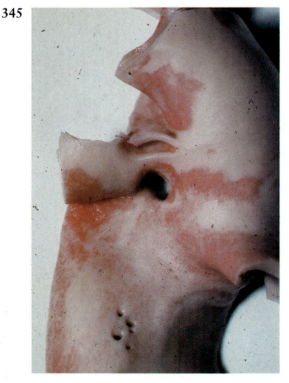

345 Baboon aorta showing red lipid in the fatty streaks produced by feeding cholesterol. (*Oil red O*)

346

346 Coronary artery from a baboon fed cholesterol. Unlike the fatty streaks in **345**, the lesion is composed largely of smooth muscle cells (top). (*H and E × 20*)

Hypertensive vascular disease and cardiac failure

Hypertensive vascular disease causes the thickening of vessels of all sizes. Arterioles in the kidney, for example, become hyaline, pink and thickened. This is called fatty hyaline change, because fat can be shown in the vessel wall. Arterioles in the suprarenal glands, the liver, the pancreas and other organs are affected, and form a useful indication that hypertension existed in life (349). Intimal fibro-elastic thickening and atherosclerosis are also aggravated by hypertension. All these changes might be regarded as a response to the increased intravascular pressure in hypertension. The left ventricular muscle also responds by hypertrophy of its fibres. This leads to relative ischaemia of the fibres, because the growth of capillary supply does not keep pace with fibre thickening. Ultimately left ventricular failure develops (347, 348).

Sometimes, in the established hypertensive, the blood pressure rises further, for as yet unknown reasons. When this happens, many vessels undergo acute necrosis, particularly those in the kidney, heart and brain. The appearance is of so-called fibrinoid necrosis; instead of the clear pink appearance of fatty hyaline change, the vessels appear smudged blue-pink and necrotic (350). Heart failure may affect both cardiac ventricles together or singly. When a ventricle fails, it can no longer maintain normal cardiac output, and the reserve ventricular volume rises. Left ventricular failure due to hypertensive disease causes a back pressure in the pulmonary vessels; plasma and erythrocytes exude into alveoli causing pulmonary oedema (351). Later, the right ventricle fails and pressure rises in the systemic veins, then oedema develops. This is the accumulation of watery fluid in the subcutaneous tissues, pleural and peritoneal cavities. The liver, spleen, kidney and other organs are engorged with blood (352, 353) and the whole syndrome is called congestive cardiac failure. Erythrocytes in the alveoli of the lung break down, and haemosiderin is taken up by macrophages (known as heart failure cells) (354, 355).

347

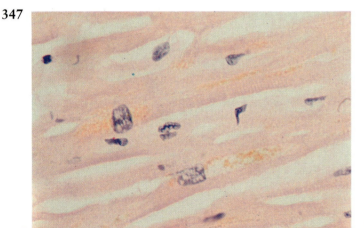

347 Normal sized fibres. Section of left ventricle showing normal sized fibres with lipochrome pigment. (*H and E × 40*)

348

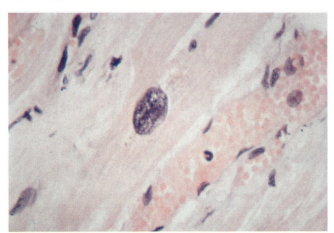

348 Hypertrophy of myocardial fibres. Section of left ventricle showing hypertrophy of myocardial fibres and nuclear enlargement. From a case of hypertensive disease. (*H and E × 40*)

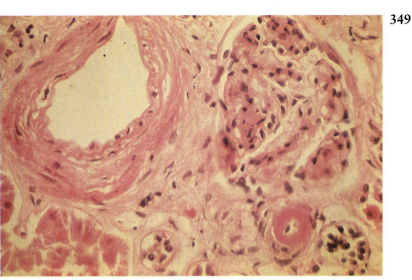

349 Hyaline change in an afferent glomerular arteriole and intimal thickening in a larger vessel (left) from a hypertensive subject. (*H and E × 10*)

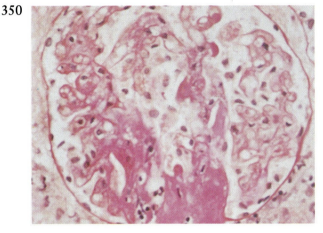

350 Fibrinoid necrosis of glomerular arterioles in malignant hypertension. The fibrinoid change extends into the tuft to involve the glomerular capillaries. (*H and E × 40*)

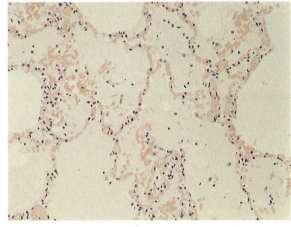

351 Lung showing acute pulmonary oedema. Pale staining oedema fluid, occasional red blood cells and macrophages in alveoli. (*H and E × 10*)

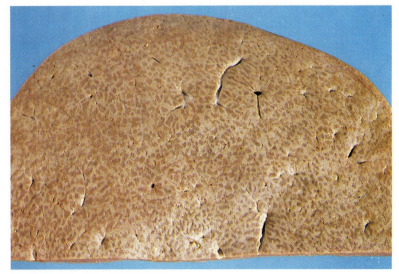

352 Congestive cardiac failure. Slice of liver from a case of congestive cardiac failure showing the characteristic nutmeg appearance. Dark and light alternating areas are present. The dark areas are due to central venous congestion.

353

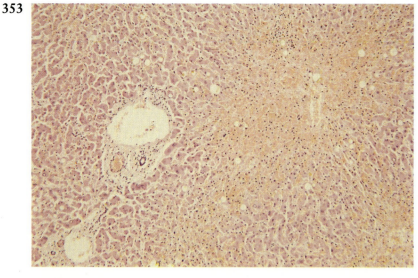

353 Congestive heart failure. Section of liver from a case of congestive cardiac failure. The centre of the lobule shows abundant red cells and some hepatocellular necrosis. (*H and E × 4*)

354

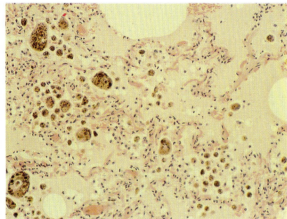

354 Brown heart failure cells in alveoli. There is some residual oedema. (*H and E × 20*)

355

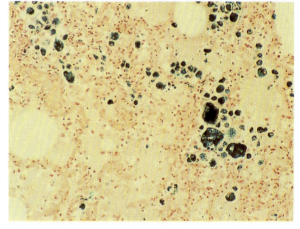

355 Heart failure cells stained to show ferric iron. (*Perls' stain × 20*)

356

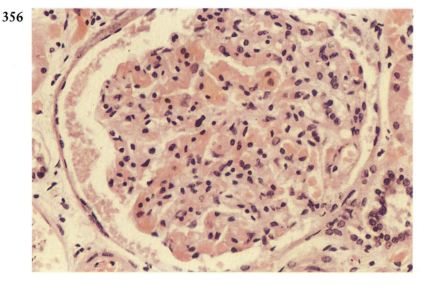

356 Congestive heart failure. Amorphous proteinaceous exudate (left) in a glomerular tuft from a case of congestive cardiac failure. Protein can be detected in the urine. (*H and E × 40*)

Allergy

Allergy means altered reaction. It is often synonymous with hypersensitivity. This is an adverse reaction which follows exposure of an animal to a second or subsequent dose of an antigen. There are many examples of hypersensitivity, such as asthma, hay fever, eczema and arteritis (359, 360). Broadly speaking, we can consider four main types of mechanism.

- *Type 1.* The antibody becomes fixed on to a reactive cell, such as a mast cell, and on further exposure to the antigen, an antigen–antibody reaction on the mast cell causes it to burst and release its granules rich in histamine. This is the basis of anaphylactic shock that may kill; it is seen after repeated antitoxin injections (for example, diphtheria and tetanus antitoxin) (357).
- *Type 2.* Here the antibody is thought to be cytotoxic; when the antibody reacts with the cell surface that bears its antigen, the cell dies. This notion underlies the concept of autoallergic diseases, where it is supposed that the body makes antibodies against its own cells; these antibodies, with complement, then destroy the individuals own cells. Hashimoto's disease of the thyroid is an example where the thyroid cells die and disappear, and the gland becomes replaced by large lymphoid foci (sometimes called struma lymphomatosa) (373).
- *Type 3.* The Arthus reaction is a rather artificial situation created by repeated injection of an antigen into the same site. After about the fourth injection, an acute swelling develops. The reaction is partly due to the formation of precipitates of antigen–antibody complexes in blood vessels, which blocks them and causes acute oedema. This, like anaphylaxis, is an acute immediate reaction (358). It is the basis of serum sickness and some forms of glomerular injury.
- *Type 4.* This type is delayed, coming on some days after a second exposure to an antigen. It is due to the effect of sensitised lymphoid cells, that go to the site and react with the antigen when it appears. It is the basis of the tuberculin reaction and of the important reaction concerned with rejection of homografts, such as

kidneys. A homograft is between two individuals of the same species. If the individuals are not genetically identical, the term allograft is used. Such grafts are rejected because the individuals have different antigens, called histocompatibility antigens. Graft rejection is mediated both by T lymphocytes and by antibodies, the latter coming into play if the individual has previously been sensitised to graft antigens. T cells are either directly cytotoxic, or liberate mediators leading to the accumulation of macrophages (362–370).

If antibodies to graft antigens are already present, hyperacute rejection occurs minutes after grafting. Antibodies bind to antigens on graft endothelium and cause complement and neutrophil damage to endothelium, leading to thrombosis. Antibodies can also cause acute delayed rejection, where vascular changes consist of the fibrinoid necrosis of arteries (361). Progressive obliteration of vessels in homografts can ultimately lead to graft failure. This is a difficult unsolved problem (371, 372).

Allergic reactions, like inflammatory reactions, consist basically of the formation of a fluid exudate mingled with cells. The following examples illustrate this.

Eczema is an acute allergic skin reaction; it may follow skin sensitisation by a variety of antigens (374).

Asthma is an allergic disorder consisting of bouts of spasm of bronchiolar muscle, making expiration difficult. Histological examination shows an infiltrate of eosinophil leucocytes in the bronchial mucosa, and thickened, hyaline fibrous tissue immediately beneath the basement membrane.

An interesting group of hypersensitivity reactions is caused by streptococcal allergy. One of these is rheumatic fever, where the joints, and more often the heart, bear the brunt of the assault. The cardiac tissues swell and contain little granulomas in the early stages (Aschoff nodules). Later, this leads to scarring and destruction of the heart valves, particularly mitral and aortic, which may become narrowed and incompetent (375–379).

Glomerulonephritis is another streptococcal allergy, where the response occurs in the glomeruli. These swell up, the capillary lumina become obliterated, many cells of Bowman's capsule proliferate to form 'crescents', and polymorphonuclear cells collect in the glomeruli. At a later stage this may cause renal failure, though the bulk of cases recover completely (380).

Sudden or unexpected infant death can occur in children aged about three months. They are often male and they tend to die in the spring or autumn of the year. The three principal postulates as caus-es are asphyxia, infection and allergy. The theory on allergy is that inhalation of cows' milk by a child that has become sensitised to it, may lead to a fatal anaphylactic shock, affecting principally the lungs. However, this is still a largely speculative view. Nowadays, the main theory of sudden infant death is that the respiratory centre is immature. However, various organisms, bacteria and viruses, have been isolated from these cases, and allergy to these may have a causative role (381, 382).

357

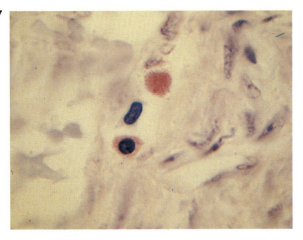

357 Mast cells occur in the connective tissues in many parts of the body. The cell nucleus is often obscured by cytoplasmic granules, as in the cell at the top. (*Solachrome cyanin × 40*)

358

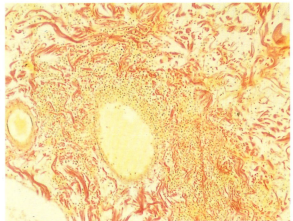

358 Arthus reaction in a rabbit. The vessel is filled with amorphous antigen–antibody precipitate and the vessel wall and surrounding tissues are infiltrated by acute inflammatory cells. (*Weigert's resorcin fuchsin ponceau S × 4*)

359

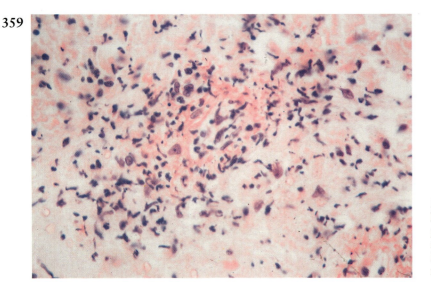

359 Acute dermal arteritis due to hypersensitivity. The vessel wall is partly destroyed, and it and the surrounding tissues are infiltrated by leucocytes, many of which are necrotic. (*H and E × 10*)

360

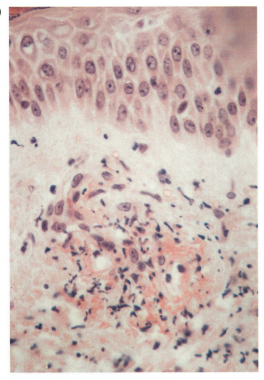

360 Dermal arteritis. A higher power view showing the epidermis (above) and the necrotic vessel wall replaced by fibrin and infiltrated by inflammatory cells. (*H and E × 20*)

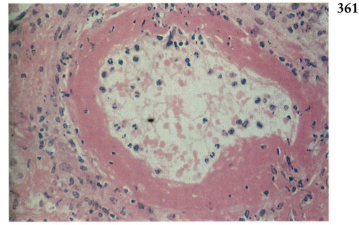

361

361 Acute late rejection showing pink fibrinoid necrosis of the artery in the graft. (*H and E × 20*)

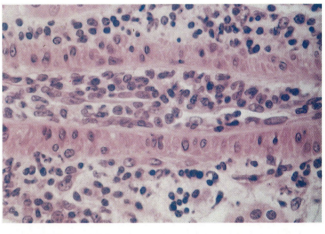

362

362 Graft rejection. T lymphocytes lifting up the arterial endothelium in graft rejection. (*H and E × 10*)

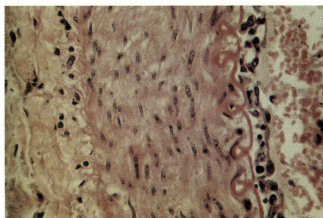

363

363 Acute rejection. Lymphocytes lying between the endothelium and internal elastic lamina in acute rejection. (*H and E × 20*)

364

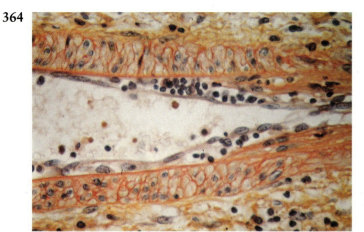

364 Subendothelial lymphocytes, elastic tissue stain. (*Weigert's resorcin fuchsin ponceau S × 10*)

365

365 Lymphocytes and foamy macrophages induced by lymphokines from the T cells lying beneath the endothelium in a rejecting graft. (*H and E × 20*)

366

366 Lymphocytes in the oedematous intima. A damaged endothelial cell has lifted off the surface, leading to the formation of a small pink thrombus on the surface. (*H and E × 20*)

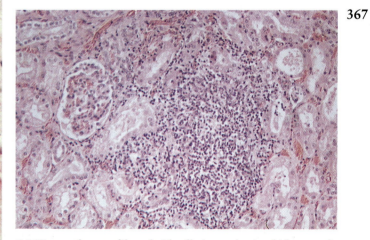

367

367 Large cluster of lymphoid cells in a rejecting kidney graft. (*H and E × 10*)

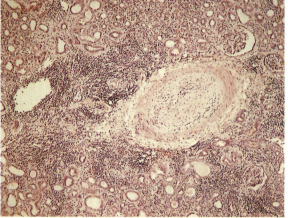

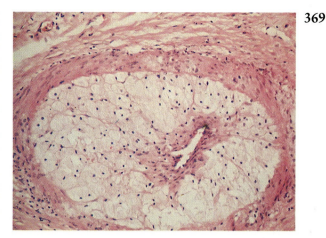

368 Chronic rejection of a renal allograft. Lymphoid cells are abundant and a vessel in the centre shows chronic obliterative changes. (*H and E × 10*)

369 Vessel from a rejecting liver graft. The intima is greatly thickened by foamy macrophages. Hyperlipidaemia in the recipient often leads to this appearance. (*H and E × 20*)

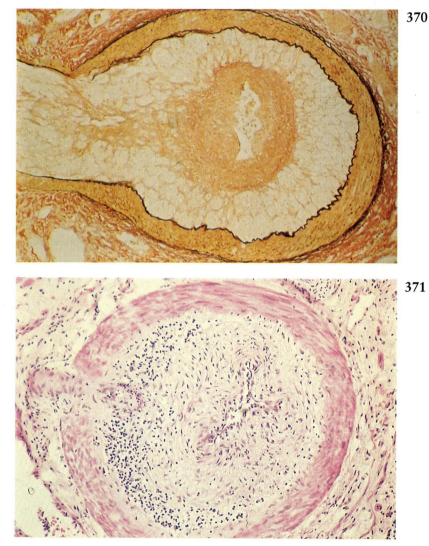

370

370 Lipid laden intimal macrophages, elastic tissue stain. The internal elastic lamina is intact. (*Weigert's resorcin fuchsin ponceau S × 20*)

371

371 Chronic vascular obliteration which is a late stage of graft rejection. Lymphocytes are scattered through the fibrous intimal thickening. (*H and E × 20*)

372

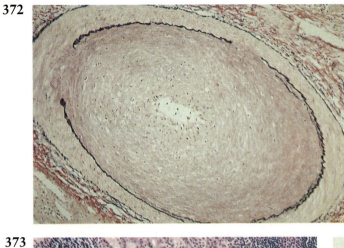

372 Chronic vascular changes in graft rejection. These lesions resemble those of atherosclerosis, but the internal elastic lamina is intact. (*Weigert's resorcin fuchsin ponceau S × 20*)

373

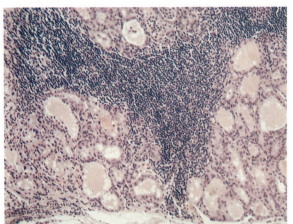

373 Hashimoto's disease. Lymphoid cells (centre) are infiltrating and damaging thyroid epithelial cells. (*H and E × 10*)

374

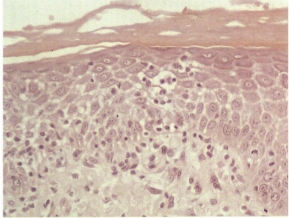

374 Section of skin from a case of eczema. Lymphocytes are present in the epidermis. Prickle cells have spaces between them. This is called spongiosis and is caused by oedema of the epithelium in this condition. (*H and E × 20*)

375

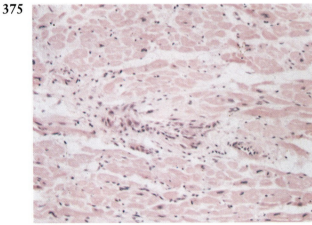

375 Aschoff nodule (centre) in the myocardium from a case of acute rheumatic fever. (*H and E × 10*)

376

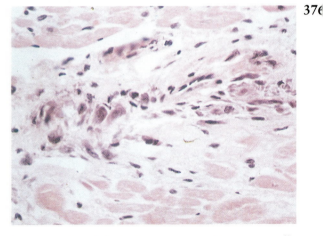

376 Aschoff nodule, high power view. Note giant cells (which usually have only a few nuclei), macrophages and degenerate collagen. (*H and E × 20*)

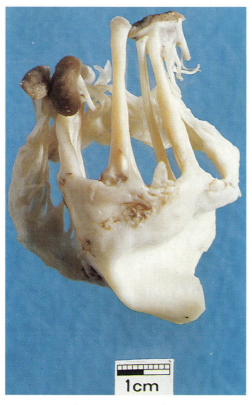

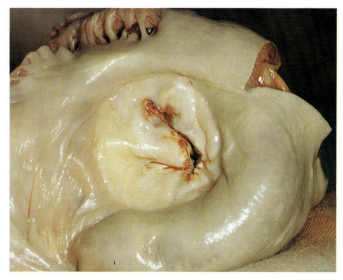

378 'Buttonhole' mitral valve. Fibrous thickening of the cusps and fusion of the commissures leads to this narrowing (stenosis) of the mitral valve orifice.

377 Surgically excised mitral valve showing white fibrous thickening of the cusps and chordae tendinae.

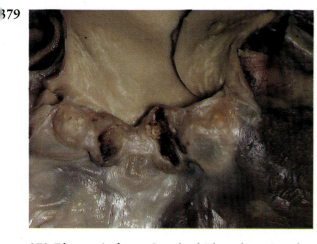

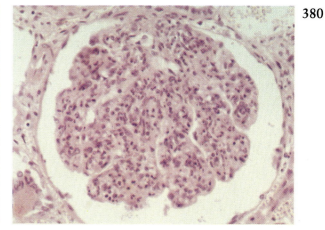

379 Rheumatic fever. Greatly thickened aortic valve cusps caused by rheumatic fever. Such fused fibrous cusps are likely to be infected by bacteria that may enter the bloodstream and produce bacterial endocarditis.

380 Glomerulus showing proliferative changes caused by antigen–antibody complexes, which lead to leucocytic infiltration of the glomerulus. (*H and E × 20*)

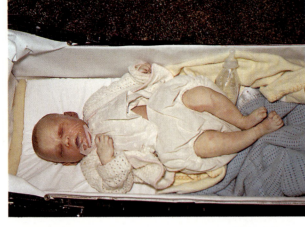

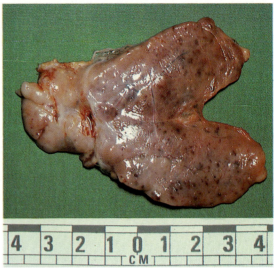

381 Typical cot death scene. The baby had been lying on its face. Note the pale pressure mark on the forehead and impressions of the neck tie. A feeding bottle is in the cot.

382 Thymus from a case of cot death showing petechial haemorrhages on the surface of the gland. Such haemorrhages are also found on other thoracic structures, such as the heart, lungs and pleura. They suggest an asphyxial component in this condition.

Intoxication

Toxic substances are abundant in the human environment, and the widespread use of all sorts of drugs in medical practice makes poisoning a common event.

Carbon monoxide in coal gas and in fumes of incomplete combustion wrecks haemoglobin as an oxygen carrier, by forming carboxyhaemoglobin. Thus tissues of people who have died suicidally or accidentally from carbon monoxide poisoning are coloured bright cherry pink (**383**).

Coal gas was often used to commit suicide. Now that it has been replaced in Britain by other forms of natural gas, barbiturates and tranquillisers have become more common suicidal agents. An interesting feature of barbiturate poisoning, and indeed of other poisons, is the tendency to cause the skin to blister, so-called toxic epidermal necrolysis. The basis of this reaction is not known (**384–386**).

Many drugs affect the liver, some destroy liver cells (for example, halogenated hydrocarbons), while others destroy bile ducts, or lead to the formation of obstructive plugs of bile pigment in canaliculi (for example, chlorpromazine) (**387–389**).

Alkaloids from plants of the genera Senecio and Crotalaria, that are found in Jamaican bush tea, have a primary effect on hepatic veins. They lead to a fibrous intimal proliferation, that may ultimately block the vessel (veno-occlusive disease of the liver) (**390**).

Aflatoxin, a product of the fungus *Aspergillus flavus*, has an interesting dual role, causing necrosis of the liver in some animals (such as birds), and neoplasms of the liver in others (such as rats and trout) (**391, 392**). The field of fungal toxins, known as mycotoxicosis, is wide ranging and developing rapidly.

Industrial poisons form an enormous subject, of which the dust diseases (pneumoconioses) are a small part. Asbestos particles, about 15 μm long, cause diffuse intra-alveolar fibrosis when inhaled into the lung (**393**). These particles become coated with haemosiderin and give a Perls' reaction. However, not all such ferrugineous bodies contain asbestos, and hence they cannot be regarded as a reliable index of asbestos inhalation in life. Asbestos also has a neoplastic promoting property, causing neoplasms of the serous membranes (pleura and peritoneum) called mesotheliomas, and it is implicated as a cause of bronchial carcinoma (q.v.).

Silicon dioxide (silica) causes focal fibrous nodules that impinge on bronchioles, and by narrowing and roughening them encourage infection, particularly with *M. tuberculosis*.

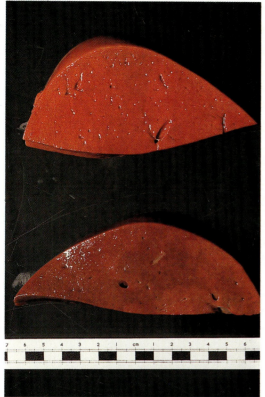

383 Carbon monoxide poisoning. Two slices of liver, the top one showing the characteristic cherry pink appearance of carbon monoxide poisoning.

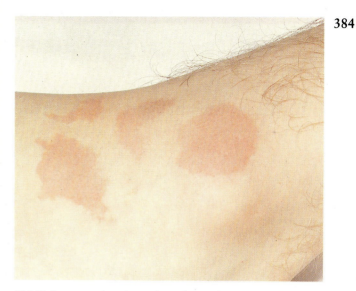

384 Pink areas of toxic epidermal necrolysis due to hypnotic drug poisoning.

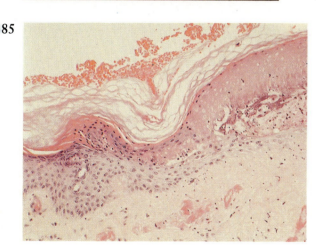

385 Toxic epidermal necrolysis of the skin. The epidermis to the right is necrotic, and a small blister is forming beneath it. (*H and E × 10*)

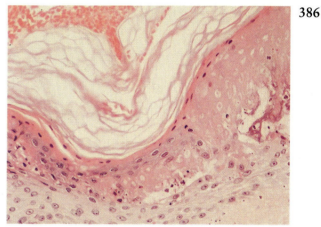

386 Toxic epidermal necrosis. Higher power view of **385**, showing loss of cell nuclei in the dead epidermis to the right. (*H and E × 20*)

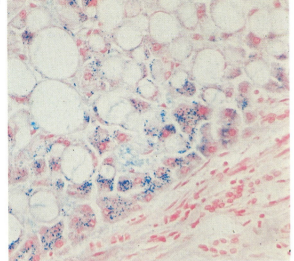

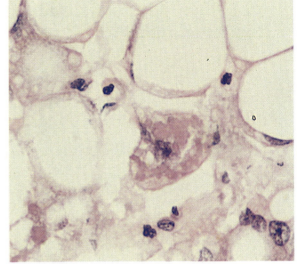

387 Fatty change in the liver of an alcoholic, showing blue haemosiderin in hepatocytes and Kupffer cells. Iron is often found in this condition. (*Perls' stain × 20*)

388 Alcoholic liver disease. Liver cells are distended with fat globules. The cell in the centre contains condensed Golgi material – Mallory's hyaline. This is not a specific feature of alcoholic liver disease. (*H and E × 40*)

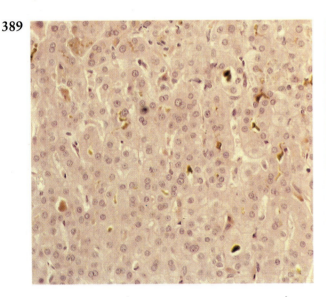

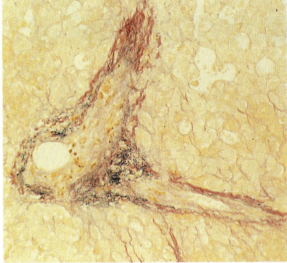

389 Section of liver showing bile plugs (brown) in canaliculi. This is caused by a variety of drugs including chlorpromazine. (*H and E × 20*)

390 Veno-occlusive disease. Central vein in a liver lobule partly occluded by collagen. (*Weigert's resorcin fuchsin ponceau S × 20*)

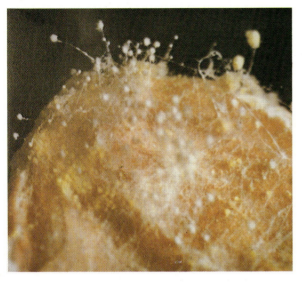

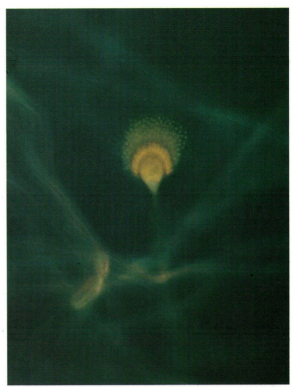

391 *Aspergillus flavus*. A peanut covered with fungal hyphae and fruiting bodies of *Aspergillus flavus*.

392 A condiophore of *Aspergillus flavus*. The green spores are born on yellow rods (sterigmata). (*Acridine orange in ultraviolet light × 10*)

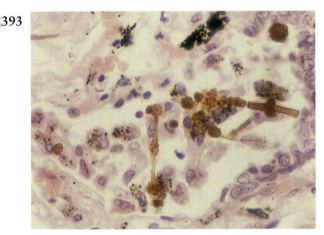

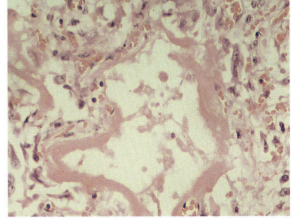

393 Yellow-brown asbestos bodies in a section of lung. (*H and E × 40*)

394 Pink hyaline membrane lining an alveolus of the lung. Such membranes occur as a result of many insults, including the inhalation of toxic gases. (*H and E × 20*)

Nutritional disorders

In the West, obesity and its attendant ills (hypertension, arthritis, lung infection, gall stones and so on) are predominant disorders, but in other parts of the world malnutrition is frequent. The effects of malnutrition are most vivid in children, whose nutritional needs are high. Nutritional deficiency is reflected particularly in rapidly growing and metabolically active structures, like bone and the liver.

Bone grows in length by the apposition of new bone, which is formed in cartilage at the epiphyseal plate (**395, 396**). Lack of vitamin D prevents calcium absorption and deposition, causing the epiphyseal plate to grow as a knob of cartilage which can be cut with a knife because it has not turned into bone (**397**). In less actively growing parts of the skeleton, where there is mature lamellar bone, rickets is indicated by osteoid seams (**398**). This is uncalcified bone matrix and is best seen in undecalcified sections of bone. Calcified bone forms a blue dye lake with haematoxylin; osteoid does not. This condition is called osteomalacia (literally bone decay) and is seen in a wide variety of conditions where there is inadequate calcium for proper bone formation.

In rickets, the epiphyseal plate is swollen. Rib epiphyses form a series of palpable nodules called a rickety rosary. Similar swellings occur in vitamin C deficiency. Here, the basic defect is the maturation of collagen, so that the epiphyseal plate is replaced by fibroblasts mingled with blood and fibrin; these are derived from capillaries that have been rendered unduly permeable by lack of vitamin C (**399**).

Vitamin A deficiency, in addition to causing defective formation of the epithelia (the cornea and skin) leads, in some animals, to new bone formation. In the skull this causes compression of cranial nerves at their emergence from foramina.

Lack of vitamin B_1 causes defective myelin formation and fatty change in the heart and other organs by affecting the intermediary metabolism (**400, 401**).

Other deficiencies, such as a lack of dietary methionine from meat, cause fatty change. This is partly responsible for the hepatic fatty change and ultimate necrosis in kwashiorkor (so-called malignant malnutrition because at least half of the children who suffer from it die). It occurs at about one year of age, when the child is weaned to a poor quality carbohydrate diet. No doubt vitamin deficiencies and parasitic infections make matters worse in these African children, but the prime disorder is a lack of protein. Carcinoma of the liver (q.v.) is a common disease in Africa, because it often arises in a cirrhotic liver that is frequently the end result of kwashiorkor.

Excess may be as bad as deficiency. The widespread practice of consuming vitamin pills and the like, may have hidden dangers. Vitamin D_3, for example, causes arterial calcification, and as much as six times the dose of this vitamin may be taken by regular consumers of certain multiple vitamin capsules (**402**).

395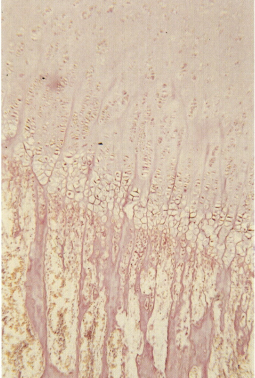

395 Normal epiphyseal plate. Columns of enlarged cartilage cells (middle) become calcified (below) as bone formation proceeds. (*H and E × 4*)

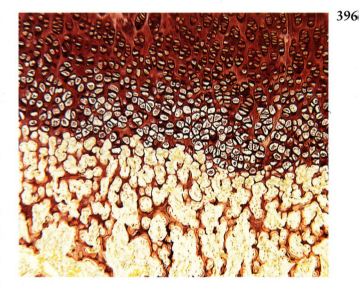
396

396 Normal epiphyseal plate showing progressive enlargement of cartilage cells from above downwards, prior to ossification of the cartilage columns. (*Weigert's resorcin fuchsin ponceau S × 4*)

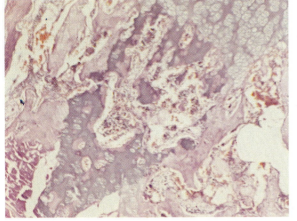

397 Rickets. An area of blue staining cartilage amongst ossifying cartilage columns. From a case of rickets. (*H and E × 10*)

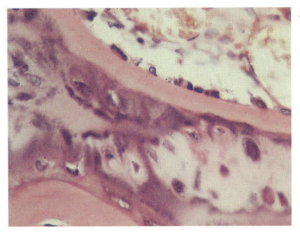

398 Pink staining osteoid seam in osteomalacia. (*H and E × 40*)

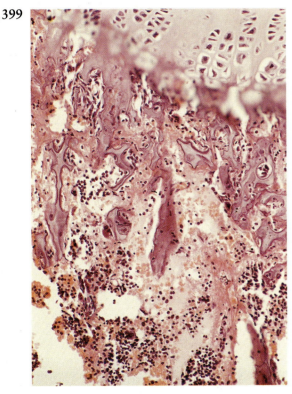

399 Vitamin C deficiency. Haemorrhage into the epiphyseal plate in scurvy (vitamin C deficiency). (*H and E × 10*)

400 Section of normal optic nerve (right) with its sheath (left) showing blue staining myelin in the nerve fibres. (*Methasol fast blue × 40*)

401 Thiamine deficiency. Optic nerve showing myelin loss. From a case of thiamine deficiency. (*Methasol fast blue × 40*)

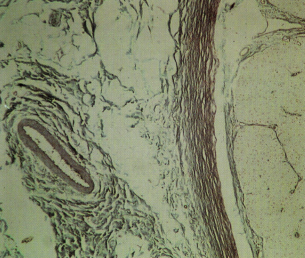

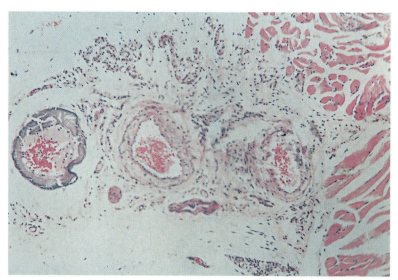

402 Blue medial calcification of an artery (left), from a rat fed vitamin D. (*H and E × 10*)

Neoplasia

Classification of neoplasia

This is one of the commonest causes of death in man. It is an uncontrolled proliferation of cells that is independent of the needs of the animal. The neoplasm may remain confined to its place of origin, when it is said to be benign, or it may infiltrate the adjacent tissues and spread to distant parts of the body (metastasis), when it is said to be malignant.

The placenta is similar to a malignant neoplasm. It grows, infiltrates the uterine wall, and pieces of trophoblast may metastasise to the lungs. After delivery, however, all trophoblastic tissue is shed or disappears; this is not so with malignant neoplasms (**403**).

Benign and malignant neoplasms can be recognised both macroscopically and microscopically. The benign neoplasms have a well formed capsule, closely resemble the parent tissue in appearance (are well differentiated), and show little evidence of cell division (few mitoses); there is no sign that the neoplasm is spreading into the adjacent tissue (**404–407**).

Malignant tumours often have no capsule, are often poorly differentiated, and can be seen to spread either into the adjacent connective tissue or along lymphatics and veins near to the neoplasm. Rapid cell division is indicated by abundant mitoses, many of which have abnormal spindles and chromosome numbers. In addition, the nuclei are hyperchromatic; they stain deeply with haematoxylin indicating abundant chromatin (**408–410**).

Neoplasms can broadly be subdivided into epithelial, mesodermal or mixed.

Benign and malignant epithelial neoplasms are common. Benign, solid epithelial neoplasms are called adenomas. When benign epithelial neoplasms project onto a surface they are called polyps; this is a non-specific term for any pathological projection, whether neoplastic or not. More accurately, one should speak of an adenomatous polyp or, if the surface is not smooth but thrown into finger-like processes, a papilloma (**416, 417**). Such polyps are common in the large intestine, on the skin and on the cervix uteri.

Malignant epithelial neoplasms are called carcinomas. These are common in the bronchus, uterus, breast, large bowel, stomach and skin. They are further specified by prefixing the kind of epithelium from which they arise; for example, squamous celled carcinoma of the skin, and columnar celled carcinoma of the colon. Because the degree of differentiation determines the prognosis to some extent, this is also indicated in a histological report.

The degree of orderliness is also important, that is, whether or not all the neoplastic islands are behaving in the same way. For example, a well differentiated squamous cell carcinoma of the skin is orderly if all the islands produce keratin. If keratin production and differentiation varies from island to island, then the neoplasm is said to be disorderly (**425**).

Grading a carcinoma is an attempt to define the prognosis from the histological appearances. Factors that are taken into account in grading vary with the observer and the type of neoplasm that is being studied. They are:

- Differentiation.
- Orderliness.
- Numbers and type of mitoses.
- Evidence of invasion or not.
- Degree of host response.

The host response varies a great deal; generally, it consists of mononuclear cells such as lymphoid cells, plasma cells and macrophages. Occasionally, other leucocytes are found, such as eosinophils and neutrophil polymorphonuclear cells. Mast cells sometimes abound in and around neoplasms; their significance is obscure.

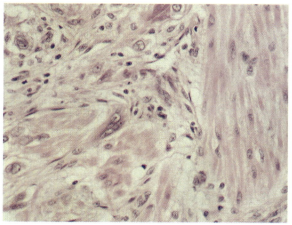

403 Syncytiotrophoblast (left) of the placenta invading the uterine wall in a normal pregnancy. (*H and E × 20*)

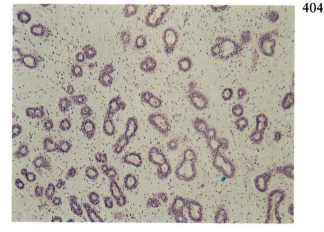

404 A benign neoplasm of the breast consisting of well formed tubules set in a cellular fibrous background. (*H and E × 4*)

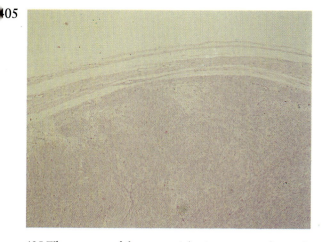

405 Fibromyoma of the uterus. A benign tumour of smooth muscle. The neoplasm has a capsule (top). (*H and E × 2*)

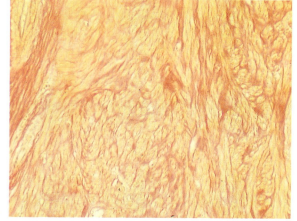

406 Fibromyoma containing smooth muscle (yellow) and bands of collagen (red). (*Weigert's resorcin fuchsin ponceau S × 10*)

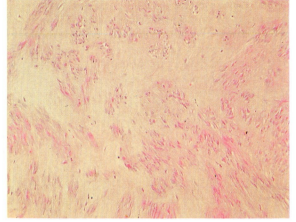

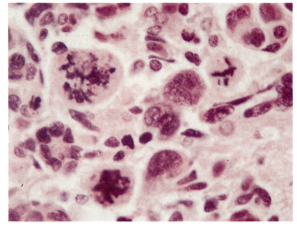

407 Fibromyomas are prone to degenerative changes. The cells of the neoplasm are replaced by hyaline pale pink collagen. (*H and E × 10*)

408 Section of a highly malignant neoplasm. The cells vary in shape and size (pleomorphism), and mitoses are abundant. Some of these are abnormal mitoses. (*H and E × 40*)

409

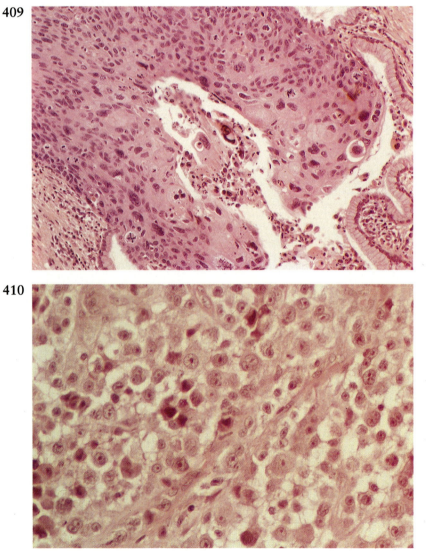

409 Pleomorphism and mitoses in a carcinoma of the uterine cervix growing into an endocervical gland lined by columnar epithelium (right). (*H and E × 10*)

410

410 Malignant melanoma which is a neoplasm of melanocyte origin. The cells are loosely attached. This lack of cohesion may be a factor in promoting spread (metastasis) of the tumour. (*H and E × 20*)

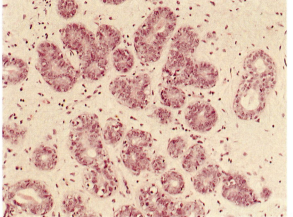

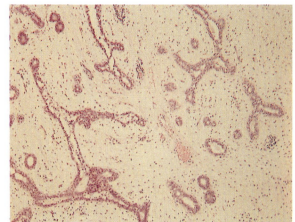

411 Adenoma of the breast – usually called a pericanalicular fibroadenoma. The cellular connective tissue stroma encircles the glandular acini. (*H and E × 10*)

412 Intracanalicular fibroadenoma of the breast. The stroma invaginates and compresses the glandular spaces. (*H and E × 4*)

413

413 The stroma of a fibroadenoma is part of the neoplasm. It may proliferate excessively. (*H and E × 20*)

414

414 Adenoma of the colon. It projects on to the surface and is called an adenomatous polyp. The normal mucosa is to the left. The tumour consists of tubules lined by columnar epithelium and is also called a tubular adenoma. (*H and E × 2*)

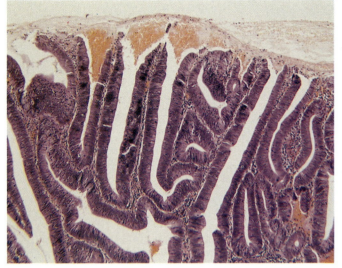

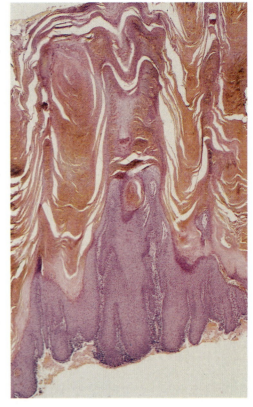

415 Villous adenoma of the colon. So called because the tumour is composed of villous finger-like processes with a vascular core. If these tumours get large they may become malignant. (*H and E × 2*)

416 Squamous papilloma of the skin. The papillae are composed of finger-like processes of epithelium capped by columns of keratin. The tumour has a sharply defined base. (*H and E × 2*)

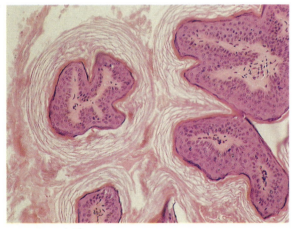

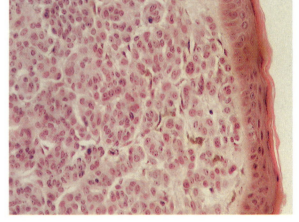

417 Squamous papilloma. Transverse section showing the epithelial papillae with a vascular core and an outer layer of keratin. (*H and E × 10*)

418 A benign neoplasm of melanocytes in the skin. The cells lie beneath the epidermis (right) and are not producing melanin. (*H and E × 20*)

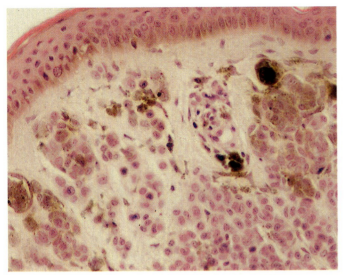

419

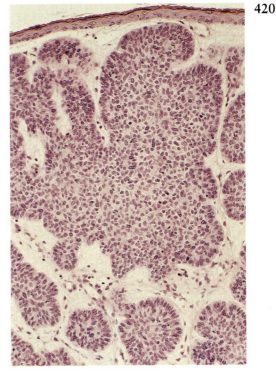

420

419 Melanocytic naevus similar to **418**. These melanocytes are producing abundant melanin. (*H and E × 20*)

420 Skin with a basal cell carcinoma in the dermis. This is a malignant tumour which usually spreads locally, destroying adjacent tissues. It rarely spreads to distant parts of the body. (*H and E × 4*)

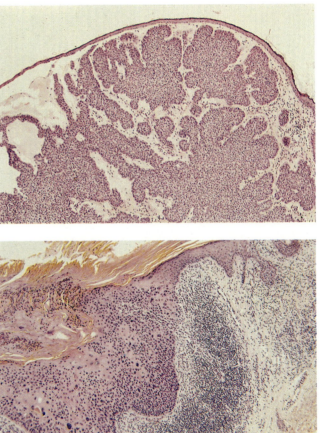

421

421 The islands of basal cell carcinoma are well defined. (*H and E × 2*)

422

422 Carcinomatous change arising within the epidermis. This is called 'carcinoma *in situ*'. The tumour has not yet spread from the confines of the epidermis. A lymphocytic reaction to the malignant process in the dermis (right) is a common feature. (*H and E × 4*)

423

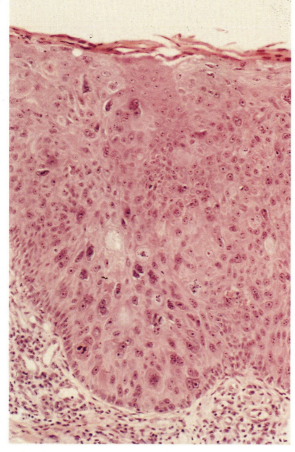

423 Epidermal carcinoma *in situ*, also called Bowen's disease, high power view. All the features of malignancy are present including hyperchromasia, pleomorphism and mitoses. (*H and E × 10*)

424

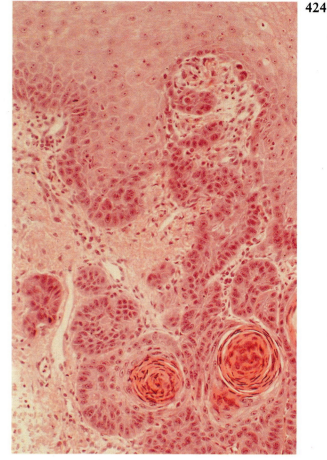

424 Skin showing a squamous cell carcinoma infiltrating the dermis. The clusters of malignant cells are producing keratin (red). These are called epithelial pearls. (*H and E × 10*)

425

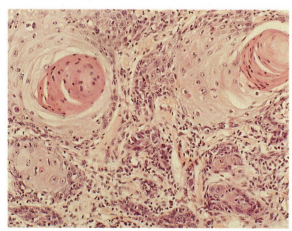

425 Squamous cell carcinoma, higher power view. Not all of the islands are producing keratin. This is a disorderly appearance suggesting a higher degree of malignancy in the tumour. (*H and E × 20*)

426

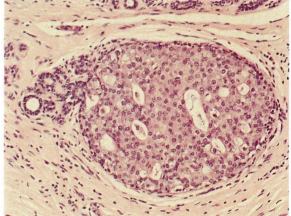

426 Carcinoma arising in a mammary duct. This is an intraduct carcinoma which has not yet invaded the surrounding stroma. This has a better prognosis than a tumour which has infiltrated the stroma. (*H and E × 10*)

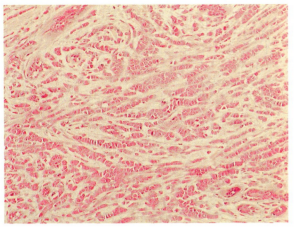

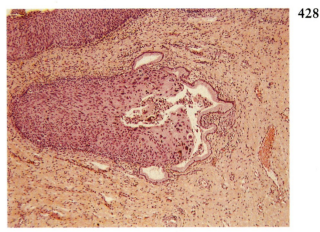

427 Lobular carcinoma. A less common variety of breast carcinoma, this is a lobular carcinoma arising from mammary lobules. Characteristically it infiltrates the stroma as columns of cells. (*H and E × 10*)

428 Carcinoma of the cervix. The epithelium (above) shows carcinoma *in situ*. In the middle of the field the tumour has invaded an endocervical gland. (*H and E × 4*)

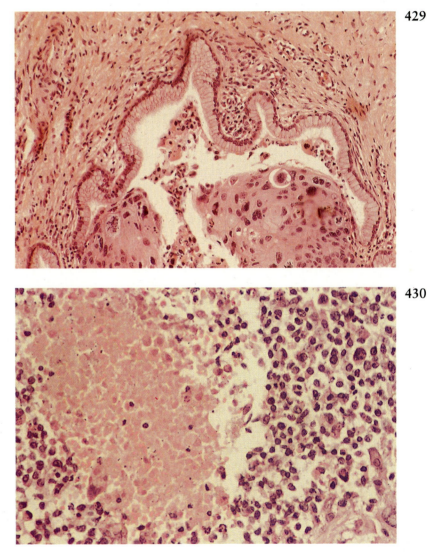

429 Cervical carcinoma invading a gland, higher power view. The tumour is anaplastic, that is, poorly differentiated. (*H and E × 10*)

430 Tumour cell necrosis. Malignant tumours often grow rapidly and outstrip their blood supply. The result is an area of tumour cell necrosis, shown pink (left). (*H and E × 20*)

Spread of neoplasia

Malignant neoplasms may spread in several ways:

- Along lymphatics by embolism or permeation.
- Along veins and capillaries.
- Along tissue spaces such as fascial planes, pleural and peritoneal surfaces.
- By direct continuity into any adjacent structure (431–434).

Carcinomas spread through the lymphatics to the lymph nodes, where the neoplastic cells grow and may replace the node (435). Some carcinomas, like those of the prostate, pancreas and tongue, tend to propagate along perineural lymphatics.

It may, however, be erroneous to think of the progress of a malignant neoplasm as occuring in stages, starting at its site of origin and slowly spreading to adjacent structures, to local lymph nodes and then to distant parts of the body. It is probably more likely that a neoplasm, from its inception, sends showers of cells into the vessels that drain it, and these are then spread over the body. Resistance mechanisms probably suppress the growth of a large proportion of these cells, particularly in organs like the spleen where metastases are not uncommon, but rarely reach a large size (436).

Bone is a favourite site for the growth of neoplastic cells from the stomach, bronchus, kidney, thyroid, prostate and breast. Most bony metastases destroy the bone (osteolytic metastases); some encourage new bone formation (osteosclerotic metastases) (439–442).

The lung is a frequent site for metastases particularly from sarcomas (q.v.). Carcinomas also frequently metastasize to the lung, and can sometimes be seen filling surface lymphatics, forming white worm-like cords on the pleural surface (lymphangitis carcinomatosa). Liver metastases are frequently seen, as one might expect, from carcinomas of the alimentary tract (the stomach, pancreas and large intestine). They spread to the liver in the branches of the portal vein.

Neoplasms in other animals are comparatively rare, compared to the incidence in man. Experimentally, neoplasms can be induced by viruses and a variety of chemical agents known as carcinogens.

431

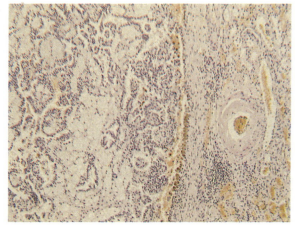

432

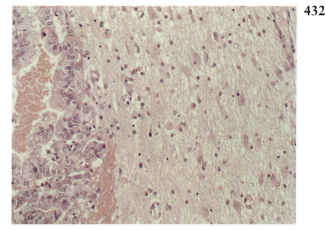

431 Carcinoma of the kidney (left). This is a well differentiated neoplasm composed of pale cells rich in glycogen. (*H and E × 4*)

432 Carcinoma of the kidney (left) which has spread to the brain (right). The brain shows a reaction of proliferating astrocytes. Even well differentiated renal neoplasms may spread to distant organs. (*H and E × 20*)

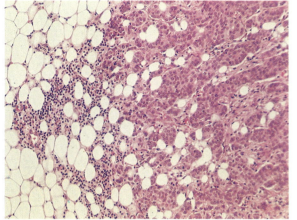

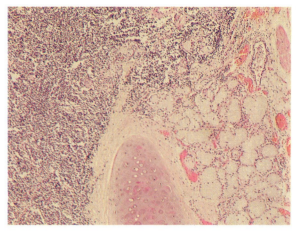

433 Carcinoma of the breast spreading locally into the adjacent fatty tissue. (*H and E × 10*)

434 Poorly differentiated carcinoma of the bronchus spreading around the bronchial wall, which contains mucous glands and cartilage (right). (*H and E × 10*)

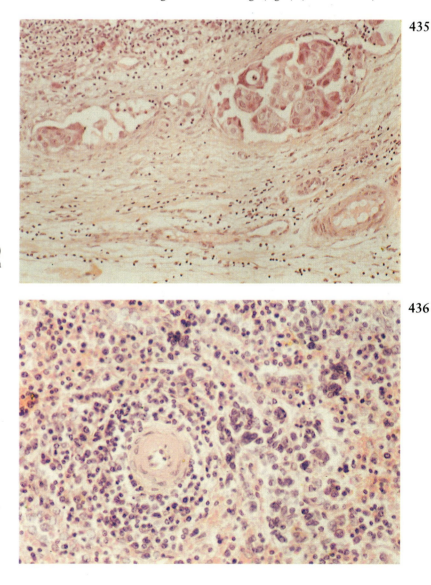

435 Islands of carcinoma cells (top) in the peripheral sinus of a lymph node. (*H and E × 10*)

436 Clumps of malignant cells in splenic sinusoids. Metastases visible to the naked eye are rare in the spleen, but microscopic deposits are not infrequent. (*H and E × 20*)

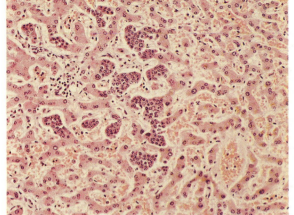

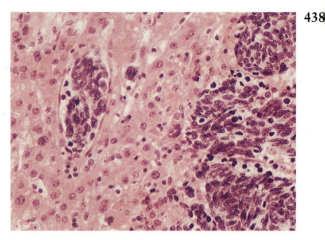

437 Malignant cells in hepatic sinusoids (left). (*H and E × 10*)

438 Oat celled carcinoma (right) of the bronchus in the liver, high power view. (*× 20*)

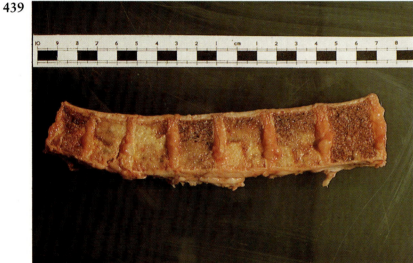

439 Carcinoma. A strip of thoracic vertebrae showing white deposits of carcinoma.

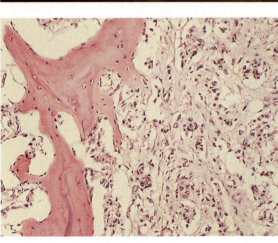

440 Islands of new bone surrounded by cells of a prostatic carcinoma. (*H and E × 10*)

441 A well differentiated prostatic carcinoma (centre) composed of small acini. New bone (right) has formed on the surface of the lamellar bone (above it). (*H and E × 10*)

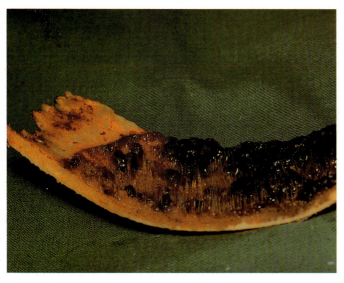

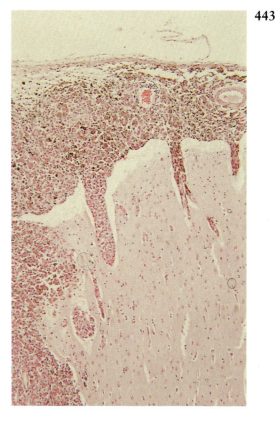

442 Spicules of new bone on the inner aspect of the skull, surrounded by dark coloured neoplastic tissue. Some neoplastic deposits are called osteosclerotic.

443 Malignant melanoma in the subarachnoid space (above) spreading into the brain (below). (*H and E × 4*)

Mesodermal neoplasia

Mesodermal neoplasms can also be classified as benign and malignant. Benign ones are common, malignant ones are rare. The benign neoplasms have a varied nomenclature, which is usually the suffix -oma (tumour) prefixed by the nature of the tissue from which it is derived, for example, osteoma, chondroma, lipoma, fibroma. Frequently, these neoplasms have more than one mesodermal component in them, and hence we have fibromyoma, osteochondroma, myolipoma, etc. (444–452).

Malignant mesodermal neoplasms are called sarcomas. They can arise in any mesodermal tissue, but usually arise from bone, cartilage and occasionally from smooth muscle; so-called osteosarcoma, chondrosarcoma and leiomyosarcoma, respectively (450, 453–456). Sarcomas differ from carcinomas in that they are richly vascular neoplasms; furthermore, the neoplastic cells themselves often form the lining of the vascular spaces. Sarcomas often spread by the veins to the lungs.

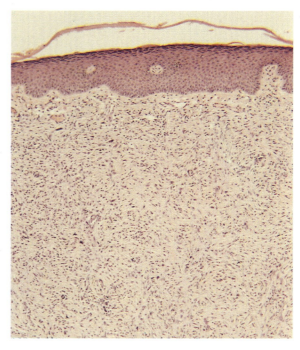

444 Fibroma of the dermis. Skin showing thickened epidermis overlying a benign connective tissue tumour which is a fibroma of the dermis. (*H and E × 4*)

445

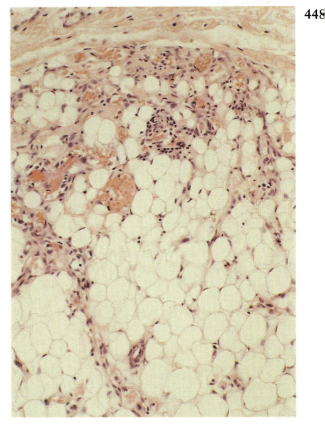

445 Dermatofibroma. Higher power view showing the swirling of cells in the neoplasm: the appearances are called storiform. (*H and E × 10*)

446

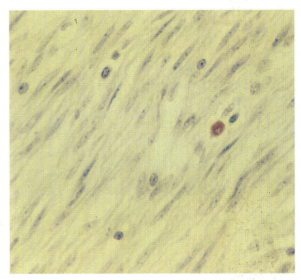

446 Fibromyoma of the uterus containing a mast cell (centre), high power view. Mast cells are often seen in and around benign tumours of connective tissue origin. (*H and E × 20*)

447

447 A benign neoplasm derived from Schwann cells (a Schwannoma). They often show this characteristic pattern of cells arranged in palisades. (*H and E × 10*)

448

448 Lipoma. The tumour is composed largely of adipose tissue cells with peripheral blood vessels. The fibrous capsule of this benign tumour is at the top. (*H and E × 10*)

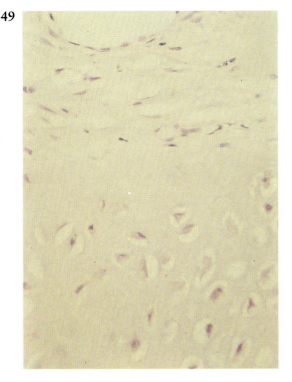

449 Section of a chondroma. This benign tumour of cartilage shows irregularly arranged cartilage cells below. (*H and E × 20*)

450

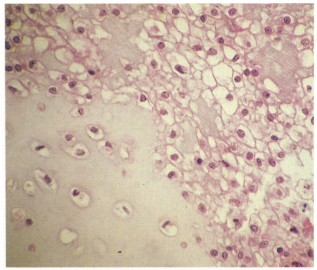

450 Tumour of cartilage. Cells on the left resemble those of a chondroma, but those on the right are pleomorphic and hyperchromatic, indicating malignant change. (*H and E × 20*)

451

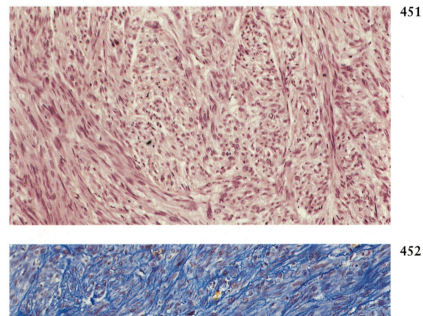

451 Benign neoplasm of spindle cells. It is sometimes difficult to decide if the cells are of fibroblastic or smooth muscle origin. (*H and E × 10*)

452

452 Fibroma. The tumour shown in **451** stained to show collagen blue. The neoplasm is therefore of fibroblastic origin: a fibroma. (*McFarlane's modification of Mallory's trichrome stain × 10*)

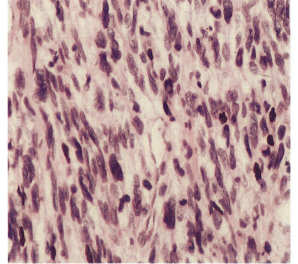

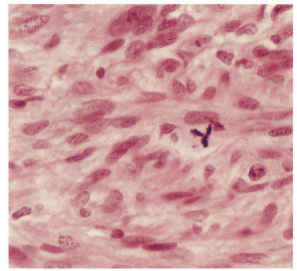

453 Malignant mesodermal neoplasm composed of pleomorphic hyperchromatic spindle cells. Immunochemical methods are necessary to decide the precise origin of this sarcoma. (*H and E × 20*)

454 Malignant mesodermal neoplasm. A high power view of the tumour in **453**, showing an abnormal tripolar mitosis (centre). (*H and E × 40*)

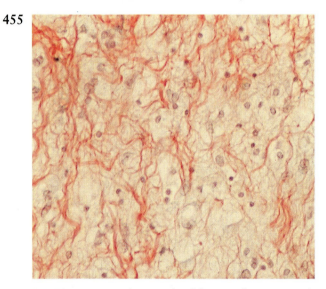

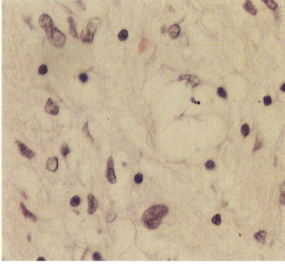

455 Liposarcoma showing the delicate collagenous pink framework of the tumour. (*Weigert's resorcin fuchsin ponceau S × 20*)

456 Liposarcoma. High power view showing a lipoblast (centre). The cell has an eccentric nucleus and fat globules in the cytoplasm. (*H and E × 40*)

Other neoplasms

Tissues, such as blood vessels, can give rise to a variety of neoplasms. Some are very common, such as the haemangioma of the skin (**457**). Sometimes several tissues appear in the neoplastic process. Such neoplasms are called teratomas. These are common tumours of the ovary, are usually benign (when they are called dermoid cysts), and may contain a variety of tissues (**458–460**).

Malignant processes can arise in haematopoietic cells. These are the various forms of leukaemia. Malignant cells may appear in the blood (**461, 462**) and may also infiltrate various organs such as the liver and spleen (**463, 464**).

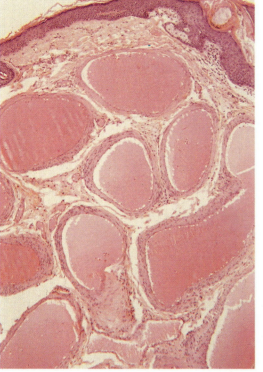

457 Haemangioma of the skin composed of dilated newly formed vascular spaces in the dermis. (*H and E × 4*)

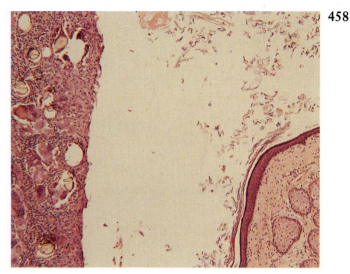

458 Dermoid cyst. Parts of the wall of a dermoid cyst in the ovary. The cyst space (centre) contains keratin flakes. Epidermis and sebaceous glands are on the right, and on the left is a granulomatous giant cell response to bits of hair and keratin. (*H and E × 4*)

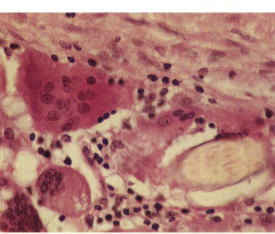

459 Dermoid cyst. Giant cells and pieces of hair (bottom right) from the wall of a dermoid cyst. (*H and E × 20*)

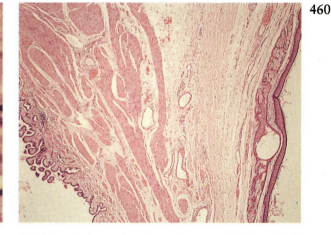

460 Dermoid cyst showing columnar epithelium (left) overlying strands of smooth muscle. Squamous epithelium (right) lies over the sebaceous glands. (*H and E × 2*)

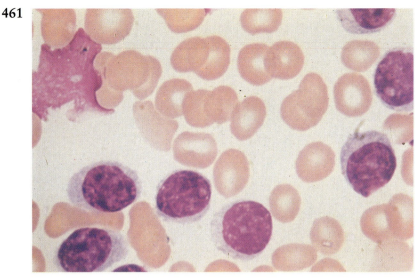

461 Chronic lymphatic leukaemia, blood film. The malignant cells are mature lymphocytes. Smudged cells (top left) are often seen. (*Leishman's stain × 100*)

462

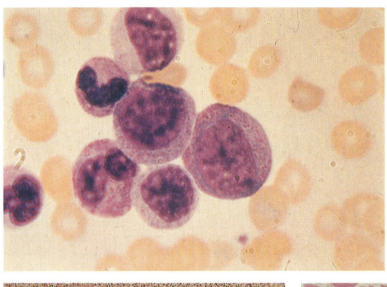

462 Chronic myeloid leukaemia, blood film. The cells are polymorphonuclear leucocytes and their precursors (cell on right). (*Leishman's stain × 100*)

463

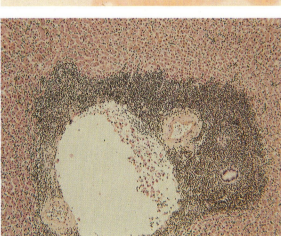

464

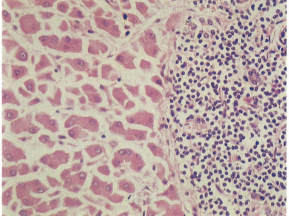

463 Lymphatic leukaemia. Portal tract in the liver infiltrated by the cells of lymphatic leukaemia. In myeloid leukaemia a more diffuse infiltration of the liver occurs. (*H and E × 4*)

464 Lymphatic leukaemia. Higher power view of the lymphoid infiltrate of lymphatic leukaemia in the liver. (*H and E × 10*)

8 Artefacts

A brief note is necessary about preparation of tissue sections in order to recognise common artefacts that may be mistaken for a pathological process.

Tissue is fixed in a dilute solution of formaldehyde, and is then dehydrated by passing it through increasing concentrations of alcohol. The tissue is then impregnated with, and embedded in, paraffin wax. The block so obtained is forced against the sharp edge of a knife in a microtome, and thin sections (about 5 μm) are sliced off the surface. These are floated on hot water, taken up on glass slides and allowed to dry. After removal of the wax by xylene and rehydration by grades of alcohol, the sections can be immersed in water and then stained with haematoxylin and eosin. After this, the process of dehydration is repeated, and the section is mounted in a plastic medium (Dystrine, Polystyrene, Xylene (DPX)) and covered with a thin cover glass.

Common artefacts are:

- Severe autolysis, due to poor fixation of pieces of tissue that are far too thick.
- Cutting artefacts, caused by a blunt knife, by a knife that is not held rigidly in the microtome, or by tough tissue such as myometrium (465).
- Floating off artefacts, caused by failure of the section to float flat on the hot water (466).
- Staining artefacts, due to either improper preparation and use of stains, or failure to remove all the wax from the section prior to staining (468).
- Various objects may become trapped between the section and the cover glass, for example, air bubbles, pollen grains and spores from the air, dust, dirt, cotton fibres and so on (469–472).
- Fixatives may lead to pigment deposition on sections, for example, formalin pigment or black deposits from mercurial fixatives (473, 474).

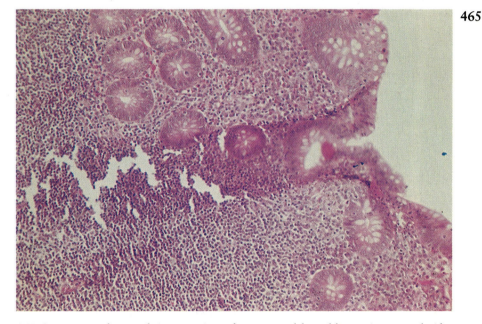

465

465 A crease and a crack in a section of gut caused by a blunt microtome knife. (*H and E × 4*)

466

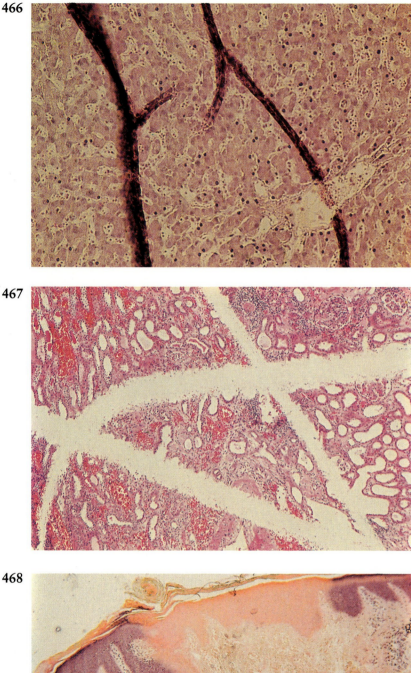

466 Creases in a section of liver. This occurs when the section does not flatten fully on hot water, usually because the water is not hot enough. (*H and E × 4*)

467

467 Scratches on this section of kidney may have a variety of causes. (*H and E × 2*)

468

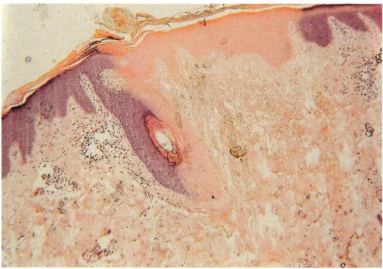

468 Section of skin. The pale pink area is where the paraffin wax has not been removed, consequently the tissue has not stained. (*H and E × 4*)

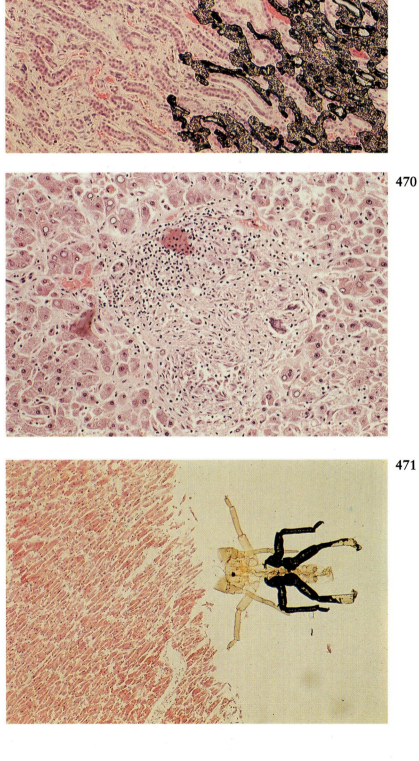

469

470

471

469 Section of kidney showing 'drying back'. The mountant was insufficient, so air crept under the cover glass (right). (*H and E × 4*)

470 Section of liver. The red blobs are squamous cells from a finger rubbed on the slide before the section was mounted. (*H and E × 4*)

471 Section of heart. An insect (right) dropped on to the slide before the cover glass was applied. (*H and E × 2*)

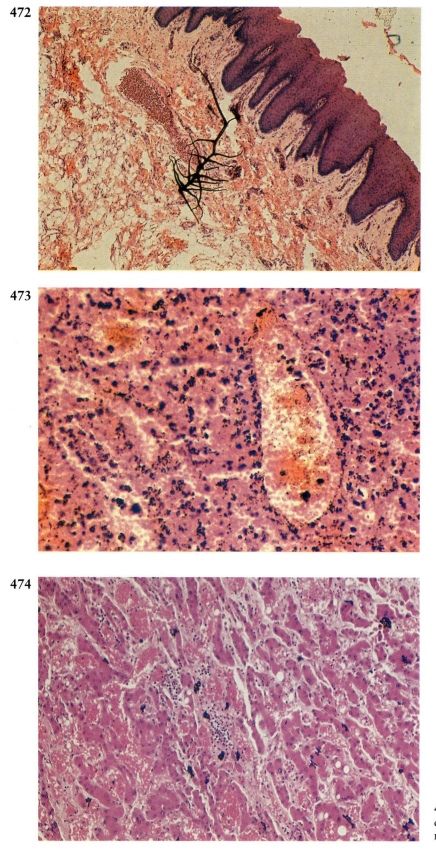

472 Pollen grain which fell on to the section before the cover glass was applied. (*H and E × 4*)

473 Black deposits of pigment from a formalin fixative obscure the histological picture. (*H and E × 4*)

474 Black deposits of pigment produced by fixation in mercuric chloride. (*H and E × 4*)

9 Glossary

Selected terms used in the text.

Abscess A localised collection of pus surrounded by granulation and often fibrous tissue.

Allograft A graft between members of the same species but of disparate genotype. Synonymous with *homograft*.

Amyloid An extracellular deposit of glycoprotein that is deposited in perivascular connective tissues and in basement membranes under certain conditions.

Anaphylaxis A sudden severe hypersensitive reaction, often associated with histamine release.

Anaplastic This describes neoplasms that are so poorly differentiated histologically that their site of origin is often uncertain. It may be difficult to decide whether an anaplastic neoplasm is a carcinoma or a sarcoma.

Anisotropic Able to deflect the plane of polarised light. Most regularly arranged substances, particularly crystals, are able to do this.

Apoptosis The death of individual cells. Literally means dropping out.

Argentaffin Having an affinity for silver salts. Argentaffin structures stain black without treatment with a reducing agent.

Argyrophil Having an affinity for silver salts. Argyrophilic structures stain black with silver salts after treatment of the tissue with a reducing agent.

Arteriosclerosis A thickening of the arteries. This is a generic term that may be applied to many conditions that lead to the thickening of arterial walls. Atherosclerosis is one form of arteriosclerosis.

Arteritis A general term used to describe inflammation in the arterial wall.

Autoallergy A state where the body makes antibodies that are toxic to some of its own cells. Autoallergic diseases, such as Hashimoto's disease, are associated with the presence in the plasma of antibody to thyroid cells. Autoimmune is sometimes used to describe such disorders.

Autolysis Self-digestion of a cell. Post mortem autolysis is a common feature of sections from human material.

Bacteraemia Bacteria in the blood. This can be detected by blood culture, but may be a transient effect that produces no outward effect on the patient.

Benign A term applied to neoplasms that are well defined, are well differentiated and do not spread to distant parts of the body or infiltrate locally.

Birefringent Synonymous with *anisotropic*.

Carcinoma A malignant neoplasm of epithelial origin.

Cirrhosis Refers to the tawny brown colour of the affected organ. It is usually applied to a fibrotic liver but has occasionally been applied to a fibrotic lung.

Cytotoxic Describes agents that damage and kill cells. Cytotoxic drugs are used to kill neoplastic cells.

Differentiation Describes the degree of resemblance of the histological appearance of a neoplasm to that of its tissue of origin.

Enteropathy A disorder of the gut. It is a general term.

Epithelioid cell A differentiated macrophage which has lost the power of phagocytosis, but can take up small particles by pinocytosis.

Exudate Fluid rich in protein and often containing cells. For example, *inflammatory exudate*.

Fatty streak Intimal thickenings that contain much lipid both within cells and extracellularly. They are characteristic of the early stage of atherosclerosis.

Fibrosis A state where collagenous and elastic fibres are deposited in excess of the normal.

Fluorochrome A dye that renders a tissue component fluorescent in ultraviolet light.

Gangrene Death of an organ, or part of it. For example, gangrene of the hand or foot.

Granuloma A localised, nodular lesion composed of cells that are usually found in chronic inflammations, for example, lymphocytes, macrophages, giant cells and eosinophil leucocytes. Variable degrees of *necrosis* may be found.

Haemosiderin A complex of ferric iron and protein that is often derived from the destruction of erythrocytes.

Heart failure cells Haemosiderin laden macrophages that are found in the alveoli of the lung in cardiac failure.

Hyperchromasia Increased colouring. Hyperchromatic nuclei are dark staining because they contain a good deal of chromatin. Nuclear hyperchromasia is often a feature of neoplasms, especially those that are malignant.

Hypoxia A state of reduced oxygen supply to a tissue, an organ or the whole body.

Infarct An area of necrosis caused by a reduction in the blood supply to an organ or tissue.

Ischaemia A state of reduced oxygenation of tissues. It can be due to depletion of haemoglobin or to vascular obstruction.

Lipochrome The complex lipid-containing substances that accumulate in cells from aged animals. It is commonly found in the heart and liver. Some think that it is derived from the breakdown of mitochondrial membranes.

Lysis A breaking up of cells. During red cell lysis haemoglobin is liberated and the cells disintegrate.

Lysosomes Cytoplasmic organelles rich in hydrolytic enzymes; their disintegration results in *autolysis*. Acid phosphatase is one of the enzymes in lysosomes, and its histochemical demonstration is a useful means of showing lysosomes.

Macrophage A large cell capable of phagocytosis. Terms such as histiocyte, monocyte, Kupffer cell and littoral cell describe macrophages in various organs.

Malignant This describes aggressive neoplasms that infiltrate into adjacent tissues and spread by the lymphatics and bloodstream to other organs. They may be poorly differentiated.

Mesenchymal Pertaining to the mesenchyme, which is a general term for the supporting tissues of the body.

Mesodermal Pertaining to the mesoderm or connecting tissues.

Mesothelium The cells that cover serous surfaces such as the pleura, pericardium and peritoneum.

Metastasis The process of spreading of a malignant neoplasm. It often leads to the formation of deposits in organs other than that in which the neoplasm arose. Such deposits are called metastases (singular – metastasis).

Microphages Polymorphonuclear phagocytes. Usually they are neutrophil cells, but eosinophils are also phagocytic.

Microvillus Delicate cytoplasmic projections, seen by electron microscopy, on the surfaces of absorbtive cells, such as in the small gut.

Mucin A term generally reserved for intracellular *mucosubstances* as in secretory epithelial cells.

Mucoid *Mucosubstance* that is found in connective tissue, cf. *mucins*, which are intracellular in epithelial cells.

Mucosubstance A general term including polysaccharide-containing substances in tissues.

Mycoplasma A genus of organisms that resemble bacteria, but do not elaborate cell walls like bacteria. They have fastidious growth requirements.

Necrolysis Death of cells accompanied by breakdown of the cells (*lysis*).

Necrosis Death of cells or tissues accompanied by visible nuclear and cytoplasmic changes.

Nutmeg liver A term describing the macroscopic mottled yellow and red appearance of the liver in chronic heart failure.

Opsonin Serum globulins that promote phagocytosis.

Osteolytic Characterised by *lysis* or destruction of bone.

Osteomalacia Defective calcification of bone, as is found in rickets.

Osteoporosis Deficiency of bony trabeculae. Common in elderly women.

Osteosclerotic Characterised by new bone formation.

Phagocytosis The property that some cells have of ingesting foreign materials such as carbon, blood pigments, etc.

Pleomorphism A variation of form. It can be used to describe nuclei or cells. Pleomorphic cells and nuclei are often a feature of anaplastic neoplasms.

Prognosis A forecast of the probable course of an illness. A good prognosis implies a likely cure and a poor prognosis may suggest death.

Purulent Associated with the formation of *pus*. For example, purulent inflammation, purulent bronchitis.

Pus The necrotic product of bacterial damage. It is composed of dead cells and bacteria.

Pyaemia A serious condition where fragments of infected material, such as pus or thrombus, circulate in the blood and block small vessels. Pyaemic emboli lead to abscess formation.

Sarcoma A malignant neoplasm of *mesenchymal* origin.

Septicaemia A situation where bacteria are multiplying in the bloodstream, causing general symptoms and signs, such as fever and shivering, which may lead to death.

Siderosis The deposition of iron-containing materials in tissues such as the lung and the liver.

Surfactant Dipalmitoyl lecithin produced by Type 2 alveolar-lining cells in the lung. It reduces surface tension and helps to maintain alveolar patency.

Teratoma A neoplasm that contains elements from several tissue components. Ovarian teratomas may contain bone, cartilage, bronchial epithelium and other elements. Teratomas may be benign or malignant.

Thrombus A laminated structure formed by blood clotting in a damaged vessel through which the blood initially flows.

Torsion The twisting of a structure. Torsion of the testis, for example, obliterates the blood supply in the spermatic cord and may cause testicular infarction.

Transudate Fluid poor in protein, such as oedema fluid, that collects in the tissue in heart failure.

Ulcer A break in an epithelial surface. Acute ulcers may heal quickly, chronic ulcers may persist for years. Ulcers may be infective or caused by trauma, irradiation or other factors.

Vascularisation The development of newly formed blood vessels in tissues. This usually occurs, in pathological states, by the growth of granulation tissue into an area of previous tissue damage.

Vasoactive Describes substances that affect the bore of blood vessels by causing either dilatation or constriction.

Prefixes

Chondro- Cartilaginous. A chondrosarcoma is a malignant neoplasm derived from cartilage.

Hyper- More, above. hypertrophy means 'more substance' and refers to an enlargement of a structure, such as a cell or an organ.

Hypo- Less, under. Hypoplasia is a reduction in the size of a cell or an organ.

Lipo- Fatty. A lipoma is a benign neoplasm of adipose tissue.

Osteo- Bony. An osteoma is a benign neoplasm of bone.

Suffixes

-itis Inflammation of a structure. Appendicitis is inflammation of the vermiform appendix. Pleuritis is inflammation of the pleura, though the term pleurisy is often preferred.

-oid Like, of a kind. So we speak of lymphoid cells when we are unable to identify the cell more precisely.

-oma A swelling or tumour. It is often applied to neoplasms, for example, osteoma, lipoma, chondroma. It can be used to describe a bruise or clot of blood, for example, haematoma.

-opathy Implies disorder. So lymphadenopathy means a disorder of lymph nodes.

-osis A condition or property. Lymphocytosis, leucocytosis and monocytosis each refer to increased numbers of the appropriate cells. Phagocytosis is a property that some cells have of ingesting material.

10 Further reading

This atlas is designed to show basic pathological processes. The following texts provide amplification of the material.

General pathology

Perhaps the best companion text to this atlas is that by Taussig. Others by Florey, McManus, Payling Wright and Perez-Tamao are older books but contain a lot of useful information and ideas. Excellent basic molecular biology of disease is contained in the book by Alberts et al.

Taussig, M. J., *Processes in pathology and microbiology* (1989) Blackwell Scientific Publications
Florey, Sir H., *General pathology* (1970) Lloyd Luke (London)
McManus, J. F. A., *General pathology* (1966) Year Book Publications, Chicago
Payling Wright, G., *An introduction to pathology* (1958) Longman's (London)
This is the earliest book on the subject and is still of great value.
Perez-Tamao, R., *Mechanisms of disease: An introduction to pathology* (1961) Saunders (Philadelphia)
Alberts, B., et al., *Molecular biology of the cell* (1989) Garland Publishing Inc. (New York and London)

Microbiology

The book by Jawetz et al. has now run into 18 editions. It is a good account of animate causes of disease.

Jawetz, E., et al., *Medical microbiology* (1991) Prentice-Hall International (London)

Immunology

There are many small books on this subject. The three below are all recommended.

Roitt, I., *Essential immunology* (1991) Blackwell Scientific Publications
Amos, W. M. G., *Basic immunology* (1981) Butterworths (London)
Turk, J. L., *Immunology in clinical medicine* (1974) Heinemann (London)

Forensic pathology

The applications of general pathology to forensic pathology are dealt with by Gresham.
Gresham, G. A., *A colour atlas of forensic pathology* (1984) Wolfe Medical Publications

Index